Surgery – Procedures, Complications, and Results

The Fundamentals of Spine Surgery

SURGERY – PROCEDURES, COMPLICATIONS, AND RESULTS

Additional books and e-books in this series can be found
on Nova's website under the Series tab.

ORTHOPEDIC RESEARCH AND THERAPY

Additional books and e-books in this series can be found
on Nova's website under the Series tab.

SURGERY – PROCEDURES, COMPLICATIONS, AND RESULTS;
ORTHOPEDIC RESEARCH AND THERAPY

THE FUNDAMENTALS OF SPINE SURGERY

TIM BACHMEIER
EDITOR

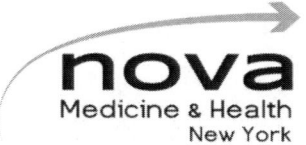

Copyright © 2020 by Nova Science Publishers, Inc.

All rights reserved. No part of this book may be reproduced, stored in a retrieval system or transmitted in any form or by any means: electronic, electrostatic, magnetic, tape, mechanical photocopying, recording or otherwise without the written permission of the Publisher.

We have partnered with Copyright Clearance Center to make it easy for you to obtain permissions to reuse content from this publication. Simply navigate to this publication's page on Nova's website and locate the "Get Permission" button below the title description. This button is linked directly to the title's permission page on copyright.com. Alternatively, you can visit copyright.com and search by title, ISBN, or ISSN.

For further questions about using the service on copyright.com, please contact:
Copyright Clearance Center
Phone: +1-(978) 750-8400   Fax: +1-(978) 750-4470   E-mail: info@copyright.com

NOTICE TO THE READER

The Publisher has taken reasonable care in the preparation of this book, but makes no expressed or implied warranty of any kind and assumes no responsibility for any errors or omissions. No liability is assumed for incidental or consequential damages in connection with or arising out of information contained in this book. The Publisher shall not be liable for any special, consequential, or exemplary damages resulting, in whole or in part, from the readers' use of, or reliance upon, this material. Any parts of this book based on government reports are so indicated and copyright is claimed for those parts to the extent applicable to compilations of such works.

Independent verification should be sought for any data, advice or recommendations contained in this book. In addition, no responsibility is assumed by the Publisher for any injury and/or damage to persons or property arising from any methods, products, instructions, ideas or otherwise contained in this publication.

This publication is designed to provide accurate and authoritative information with regard to the subject matter covered herein. It is sold with the clear understanding that the Publisher is not engaged in rendering legal or any other professional services. If legal or any other expert assistance is required, the services of a competent person should be sought. FROM A DECLARATION OF PARTICIPANTS JOINTLY ADOPTED BY A COMMITTEE OF THE AMERICAN BAR ASSOCIATION AND A COMMITTEE OF PUBLISHERS.

Additional color graphics may be available in the e-book version of this book.

Library of Congress Cataloging-in-Publication Data

Names: Bachmeier, Tim, editor. Title: The fundamentals of spine surgery / Tim Bachmeier, editor.
Description: New York : Nova Science Publishers, [2020] | Series: Surgery - procedures, complications, and results; orthopedic research and therapy | Includes bibliographical references and index. | Summary: "The Fundamentals of Spine Surgery first aims to investigate the efficacy of several therapeutic modalities in the modern treatment of spinal pathologies. Following this, the authors aim to estimate fusion by 3D CT scan in XLIFs applied in adult lumbar deformities, evaluating the clinical results related to fusion. The safety and effectiveness of minimally invasive-transforaminal lumbar interbody fusion in the treatment of lumbar degenerative spondylolisthesis is evaluated, highlighting the steps and technical procedures of this operation as well as its short and long-term outcomes. In the closing study, the authors compare the effectiveness of spino-pelvic parameters in minimally invasive posterior lumbar interbody fusion and traditional posterior open approach in the treatment of a prospective randomized series of high-grade adult isthmic spondylolisthesis"-- Provided by publisher.
Identifiers: LCCN 2020041697 (print) | LCCN 2020041698 (ebook) | ISBN 9781536185706 (paperback) | ISBN 9781536187410 (adobe pdf)
Subjects: LCSH: Spine--Surgery. Classification: LCC RD768 .F78 2020 (print) | LCC RD768 (ebook) | DDC 617.4/71--dc23
LC record available at https://lccn.loc.gov/2020041697
LC ebook record available at https://lccn.loc.gov/2020041698

Published by Nova Science Publishers, Inc. † *New York*

CONTENTS

Preface		vii
Chapter 1	Cellular Technologies in the Treatment of Orthopaedic Spine Pathologies *Bejan A. Alvandi, Connor Willis-Hong, Kelly Wun and Vivek Mohan*	1
Chapter 2	Fusion Rate after LLIF Procedures in Lumbar Adult Deformities: The State of Art *Andrea Perna, Alessandro Ramieri, Luca Ricciardi, Luca Proietti, Massimo Miscusi, Georgios Bakaloudis, Domenico Alessandro Santagada, Francesco Ciro Tamburrelli, Antonino Raco and Giuseppe Costanzo*	55
Chapter 3	Posterior Fusion in Degenerative Spondylolisthesis: The Role of the Minimally Invasive Transforaminal Approach (MI-TLIF) *Alessandro Ramieri, Giorgio Rossi, Omar Alshafeei, Vincenzo Barci and Giuseppe Costanzo*	89

Chapter 4	Minimally Invasive vs Conventional Open Posterior Lumbar Interbody Fusion in the Treatment of High-Grade L5 Isthmic Spondylolisthesis *Alessandro Ramieri, Massimo Miscusi, Sokol Trungu, Stefano Forcato, Amedeo Piazza, Antonino Raco and Giuseppe Costanzo*	**119**
Index		**135**

PREFACE

The Fundamentals of Spine Surgery first aims to investigate the efficacy of several therapeutic modalities in the modern treatment of spinal pathologies.

Following this, the authors aim to estimate fusion by 3D CT scan in XLIFs applied in adult lumbar deformities, evaluating the clinical results related to fusion.

The safety and effectiveness of minimally invasive-transforaminal lumbar interbody fusion in the treatment of lumbar degenerative spondylolisthesis is evaluated, highlighting the steps and technical procedures of this operation as well as its short and long-term outcomes.

In the closing study, the authors compare the effectiveness of spino-pelvic parameters in minimally invasive posterior lumbar interbody fusion and traditional posterior open approach in the treatment of a prospective randomized series of high-grade adult isthmic spondylolisthesis.

Chapter 1 - In recent years, biologics have found increasing utility and acceptance in the field of orthopaedic spine surgery. These novel cellular technologies offer promising results as primary and adjuvant treatments for patients with a variety of bone and soft tissue spinal pathologies. Understanding how these therapies function in reducing pain, increasing function, and altering disease progression may have significant clinical implications. Stem cells - both autograft and allograft - are undifferentiated cellular precursors with regenerative capacity. These cells have the potential to restore form and function in degenerative disease with limited biologic plasticity. Additionally, stem cells potentially enhance fixation by accelerating bone healing after surgical stabilization of the spine. Platelet-rich plasma (PRP) is serum-derived growth factor concentrate which has shown clinical benefit in targeted musculoskeletal disease treatment. PRP helps to slow - and possibly reverse - degenerative spine disease through cell and extracellular matrix proliferation. Exosomal injections deliver extracellular vesicles, on the order of 1,000 times smaller than stem cells, to target areas where they are endocytosed by receptor cells. Exosomes contain growth factors, signalling lipids, and RNAs sequences shown to stimulate osteogenesis, reduce cellular apoptosis, and improve pain scores. This chapter aims to investigate the efficacy of these therapeutic modalities in the modern treatment of spinal pathologies.

Chapter 2 - Purpose: In few studies, fusion rate in XLIF, assessed by CT scan, ranged between 85 and 93%. Aims of the authors' study were: - estimate fusion by 3D CT scan in XLIFs applied only in adult lumbar deformities; - evaluate clinical results related to fusion. Materials and Methods: 193 XLIFs (147 titanium, 51peeks) performed in 79 adult degenerative lumbar scoliosis and 44 spondylolisthesis were evaluated by 3D CT scan at least 1 yr follow-up, distinguishing complete fusion (F), probably fusion (PF) and pseudoarthrosis (P), as well as subsidence and/or mobilization. Clinical results on VAS and ODI were compared in relation to the degree of fusion. Different bone grafts were used: bovine bone mineral and collagen; calcium phosphate granules or paste; paste of demineralized bone matrix. Results: The authors recorded 75% of F, 19% of PF and 6% P. Pseudoarthrosis involved 7 titanium and 6 PEEK cages. Particularly exposed to subsidence or settling were middle cages in 3-level XLIFs. The worst clinical condition concerned pseudoarthrosis with loss of correction. Conclusions: The fusion rate in the authors' case series, consisting of only adult deformities, at one year follow-up, was lower than those reported in the literature. Pseudoarthrosis, cage settling and loss of lumbar lordosis correction were factors that negatively affected the authors' clinical outcomes.

Chapter 3 - There are numerous surgical options for patients with LDS (Lumbar Degenerative Spondylolisthesis). The operations are chosen accordingly to the surgeon's experience and his/her personal conduct and can be performed in an open or minimally invasive way. "What type of surgery" argument is still highly controversial and debated. To date, a paucity of literature exists to evaluate safety and effectiveness of MI-TLIF (Minimally Invasive - Transforaminal Lumbar Interbody Fusion) in the treatment of LDS. The purpose of this paper is to show, in detail, the steps and technical procedures of this operation, as well as evaluating its short and long-term outcomes. MI-TLIF, combined with Percutaneous Placement of Pedicle Screws and Rods, was performed in a cohort of 23 patients with LDS. In each patient, the level of anterolisthesis and the presence of a lumbar stenosis and/or herniated disc were verified. Operative data (operative time, estimated blood loss), length of hospitalization and complications were assessed. In the pre-operative and in the FUP (follow-up), VAS (Visual Analogue Scale) and ODI (Oswestry Disability Index) were calculated. In the FUP Radiographic check, MacNab score and Patient Satisfaction were also evaluated. The total mean operative time was 170 ± 22.3 minutes and the mean blood loss was 205 ± 38.2 ml. The mean duration of hospitalization was 5 ± 1.6 days. No patient needed transfusion and none had infections. The total acquired neurological deficit rate was 13%. In the pre-operative and in the FUP, registered scores were compared using t-test. Statistically significant differences emerged in the VAS back ($p = 0.045$), in the VAS leg ($p = 0.018$) and in the ODI ($p = 0.013$). Furthermore, in the FUP the Radiographic check showed no implant problems and MacNab criteria had a good outcome in 78.3% of the patients. Eighteen patients would undergo this surgical operation again. MI-TLIF may provide effective short and long term clinical-functional improvements in patients with LDS. Minimally invasive surgery guarantees a minimized tissue disruption and decreases the length of hospitalization and functional recovery times. Despite the possible post-operative root suffering, the technique can be considered safe and effective as shown in more than 80% of the authors' patients.

Chapter 4 - Purpose: To compare the effectiveness and changes of the spino-pelvic parameters between the minimally invasive PLIF and traditional posterior open approach in the treatment of a prospective randomized series of high-grade adult isthmic spondylolisthesis (HGISL). Material and Methods: Two homogeneous groups of 14 adult patients with a painful high-grade isthmic L5 spondylolisthesis (Meyerding III or IV) were operated by open (group A) and minimally invasive PLIF (MISS group B). L4-S1 instrumentation and L5-S1 interbody fusion were realized. Deformities were classified according to the SDSG, measuring slippage, slip angle, thoracic kyphosis (TK), lumbar lordosis (LL), sagittal vertical axis (SVA), pelvic tilt (PT). A PT value $\leq 30°$ was assumed as a condition of balanced pelvis. Clinical evaluation was based on the back and leg VAS, ODI and SF36. Results: Mean age was 24 (range 19-39), with F:M ratio 2.5:1. Seven deformities were type 7 and 21 type 8. The authors had 7% of early major neurological complications, Blood loss was greater in group A (p 0.037), as the hospital lenght (p = 0.02). At follow-up (mean 29.4, range 24-42), radiographic and clinical parameters overall improved ($p < 0.05$), without significant differences between groups ($p > 0.05$). The PT decreased below 30° degrees in 9 type 8 HGISL. The SVA moved slightly forward and LL showed a little reduction ($p > 0.05$). A slip angle >10° was related to the worst clinical follow-up painful condition ($p < 0.03$). Conclusion: As in other spinal diseases, the posterior MISS seems to be non-inferior to open approach in the HGISL surgical care. MISS was better in relation to the estimated blood loss and hospital lenght. Changes of spino-pelvic parameters were observed in both procedures, but further studies will be required to demonstrate a clear correlation between radiological and clinical results. Data showed that the authors' estimated parameters did not significantly affect the clinical outcomes as measured at the last follow-up, except for the slip angle.

In: The Fundamentals of Spine Surgery
Editor: Tim Bachmeier

ISBN: 978-1-53618-570-6
© 2020 Nova Science Publishers, Inc.

Chapter 1

CELLULAR TECHNOLOGIES IN THE TREATMENT OF ORTHOPAEDIC SPINE PATHOLOGIES

Bejan A. Alvandi[1], *MD, Connor Willis-Hong*[2],
Kelly Wun[1], *MD and Vivek Mohan*[2,*], *MD*

[1]Department of Orthopaedic Surgery, Feinberg School of Medicine,
Northwestern University, Chicago, IL, US
[2]Orthopaedic Spine Institute. Chicago, IL, US

ABSTRACT

In recent years, biologics have found increasing utility and acceptance in the field of orthopaedic spine surgery. These novel cellular technologies offer promising results as primary and adjuvant treatments for patients with a variety of bone and soft tissue spinal pathologies. Understanding how these therapies function in reducing pain, increasing function, and altering disease progression may have significant clinical implications. Stem cells - both autograft and allograft - are undifferentiated cellular precursors with regenerative capacity. These cells have the potential to restore form and function in degenerative disease with limited biologic plasticity.

---

[*] Corresponding Author's E-mail: spine.vivek@gmail.com.

Additionally, stem cells potentially enhance fixation by accelerating bone healing after surgical stabilization of the spine. Platelet-rich plasma (PRP) is serum-derived growth factor concentrate which has shown clinical benefit in targeted musculoskeletal disease treatment. PRP helps to slow - and possibly reverse - degenerative spine disease through cell and extracellular matrix proliferation. Exosomal injections deliver extracellular vesicles, on the order of 1,000 times smaller than stem cells, to target areas where they are endocytosed by receptor cells. Exosomes contain growth factors, signalling lipids, and RNAs sequences shown to stimulate osteogenesis, reduce cellular apoptosis, and improve pain scores. This chapter aims to investigate the efficacy of these therapeutic modalities in the modern treatment of spinal pathologies.

INTRODUCTION

Platelets, or thrombocytes, are cells derived from megakaryocytes through a series of progenitor cells and are traditionally known for its critical role in the generation and propagation of blood clots. Physiologic platelet function is to promote hemostasis through platelet adhesion, activation, and aggregation of additional platelets in response to vascular injury. In conjunction with factors involved in the clotting cascade, specifically ionized calcium and thrombin, platelet activation is mediated through endogenous factors. Upon activation of platelets, growth factors and cytokines are released to promote inflammation, cellular recruitment, and cellular proliferation to facilitate repair and healing of injury. This mechanism is critical for wound healing and tissue repair.

Platelet-rich plasma (PRP) is an autologously-derived blood concentrate of platelets isolated through a centrifugation process of peripheral blood. The concept of PRP was first described in the 1970s, followed by its clinical use a decade later in oral and maxillofacial surgery. Eventually, periodontics, plastic surgery, urology, sports medicine, and orthopaedic surgery followed suit in development of specialty-specific applications of PRP. In orthopaedics, PRP has gained popularity since its introduction particularly in knee osteoarthritis, rotator cuff pathologies, anterior cruciate ligament repair, and patellar and Achilles' tendinopathies (Hussain, Johal, and Bhandari 2017; Delgado et al. 2019; Kenmochi 2020; Wasterlain et al.

2013; Noh et al. 2018). Though there is growing evidence on the utility and efficacy of PRP injections in musculoskeletal pathologies, outcomes and current clinical utility of its use is yet to be fully elucidated (Hussain, Johal, and Bhandari 2017; Salamanna et al. 2015). In spine surgery, biologics have gained popularity, specifically rh-BMP-2 in lumbosacral spinal fusions. However, use of rh-BMP-2 is not without its risks including ectopic bone formation, radiculopathy, retrograde ejaculation, graft subsidence, and osteosarcoma (Greene and Hsu 2019; Weiss 2015). Cost represents another limitation to the use of BMP in spine surgery with direct costs averaging $14,000 compared to the average cost of $800 for single PRP injection (Hussain, Johal, and Bhandari 2017; Louie, Hassanzadeh, and Singh 2014; A. Jain et al. 2020). Given the current limitations to the presently available orthobiologics in spine surgery, the clinical application of PRP in spine surgery is yet to be fully elucidated and represents an appealing autologous biologic with potential in the field of spine surgery.

PRP: Production, Characteristics, and Mechanism of Action

PRP is derived from autologous blood that is centrifuged to separate the various components contained within the patient's whole blood. Following centrifugation, red blood cells (RBCs) constitute the densest layer following centrifugation representing approximately 45% of the blood volume, followed by the buffy coat (< 1% by volume), then plasma (55% by volume). The buffy coat consists of platelets and white blood cells in the PRP preparation. Further concentration and separation of blood components yields platelet-rich and platelet-poor layers (Hall et al. 2009). Optimal concentrations of platelets is 3 – 5 times the whole blood concentration of platelets, where PRP platelet concentrations greater than 5 times that of whole blood can inhibit healing.

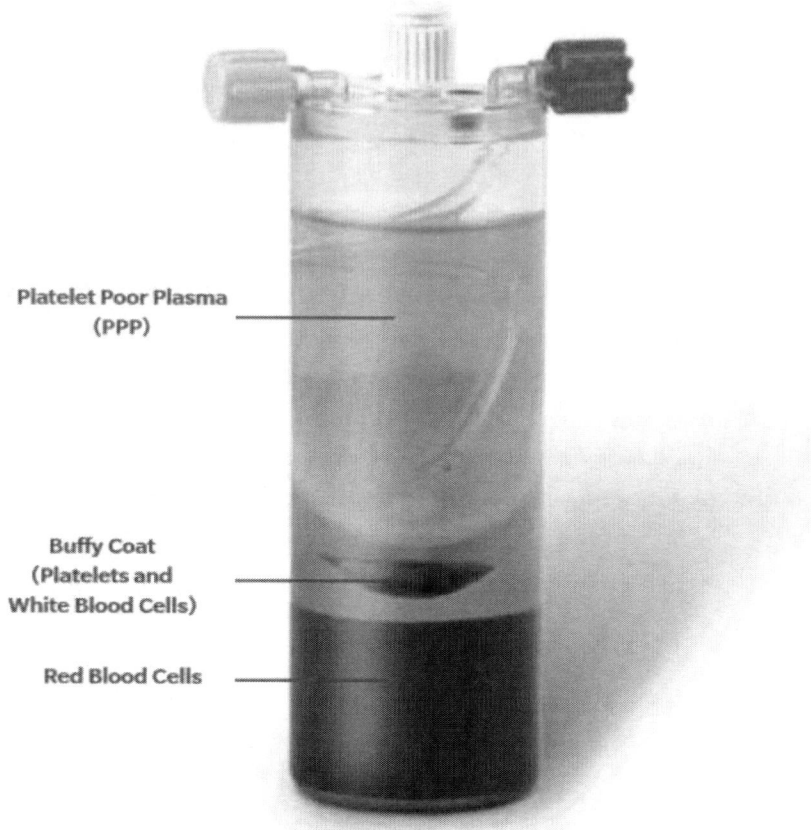

Figure 1. Sample of centrifuged blood depicting the separated layers. Platelets are isolated from the buffy coat (Hall et al. 2009).

Four formulations of PRP can be prepared: activated, non-activated, leukocyte-rich, and leukocyte-poor (Yaari, Dolev, and Haviv 2019). Activation of PRP can be facilitated through exogenous or endogenous factors following administration. Calcium chloride or thrombin combined with PRP results in immediate activation of PRP and platelets to release growth factors and initiate clotting.

Endogenously-derived factors, such as tendon-derived collagen, have been shown to be capable of slow activation of PRP Following activation of platelets in the PRP preparation, the release of cytokines and growth factors is hypothesized to facilitate improved healing and bone regeneration.

In terms of wound healing, leukocytes in leukocyte-rich PRP stimulate pro-inflammatory cascades that may counter the effects of healing and tissue regeneration by growth factors, therefore exclusion of leukocytes to produce leukocyte-poor PRP is may optimize wound healing potential (S. Z. Wang et al. 2018; Simental-Mendia et al. 2018).

Autologous platelets contain growth factors including platelet-derived growth factor (PDGF), transforming growth factor beta (TGF-B), vascular endothelial growth factor (VEGF), insulin-like growth factor 1 (IGF-1), epidermal growth factor (EGF), connective tissue growth factor (CTGF), and fibroblast growth factor 2 (FGF-2). These growth factors promote cellular regeneration, mitogenesis, angiogenesis, and therefore healing through cellular pathways that promote and upregulate cellular growth and proliferation. For example, PDGF activation of PDGF receptor (PDGFR) has been shown to increase cell signaling pathways that can promote bony fusion (Kinoshita et al. 2020).

Table 1. Growth factors and growth factor function released following platelet activation

Growth Factor	Function
PDGF	Osteoblast proliferation & differentiation, promote bony fusion, fibroblast proliferation, angiogenesis
TGF-B	Fibroblast proliferation, stimulates collagen type 1 and type 3, angiogenesis
VEGF	Angiogenesis, fibroblast proliferation
IGF-1	Myoblast & fibroblast activation, induction of osteoblast matrix secretion
FGF-2	Endothelial cell proliferation, angiogenesis

In vitro studies of PRP in combination with bone mesenchymal stem cells (BMSC) have demonstrated accelerated bone regeneration and increased neovascularization compared to controls and PRP-alone, or

BMSC-alone along with increased cellular proliferation and osteogenic activity (Salamanna et al. 2015; Yamakawa et al. 2017). These studies provide preliminary evidence of the potential utility of PRP for orthopaedic applications.

CURRENT INDICATIONS IN SPINE

Low Back Pain

Low back pain (LBP) is a very common condition with approximately prevalence of 7.3% activity-limiting LBP with a 1-month prevalence of 23% with a greater prevalence in females than males (Akeda et al. 2019). Etiology of low back pain is broad and includes discogenic pain, degenerative disc disease, disc herniation, facet arthropathy, ligamentum flavum hypertrophy, ossification of the posterior longitudinal ligament, spinal stenosis, and spondylolisthesis.

Although the specific pathogenesis of discogenic low back pain is not exactly known, changes in the composition of the intervertebral disc is implicated. The present biochemical understanding of intervertebral disc changes includes decreases in proteoglycan and type II collagen followed by decreased water content and increased fraction of type 1 collagen (Akeda et al. 2019). Disc degeneration is radiographically characterized by hypointensity on T2-weighted MRI and biologically characterized by degeneration of the extracellular matrix of the disc, which consists of decreased proteoglycan matrix and decreased water content of the nucleus pulposus and annulus fibrosus. These features are characteristic of disc degeneration and these degenerative changes can lead to structural disruptions in the intervertebral disc causing pain (Akeda et al. 2019; Pirvu et al. 2014; Baig et al. 2020).

The process of disc degeneration is hypothesized to be caused by tears in the annulus fibrosus followed by loss of disc height and disc resorption. Intradiscal injection of PRP represents a potential intervention for management of intervertebral disc degeneration and discogenic back pain and *in vivo* studies have demonstrated partial restoration of disc height and disc hydration (Monfett et al. 2016; Mohammed and Yu 2018). For the treatment of disc herniation, PRP has been shown to promote annulus fibrosis repair through increased matrix production and cell proliferation and viability (Pirvu et al. 2014).

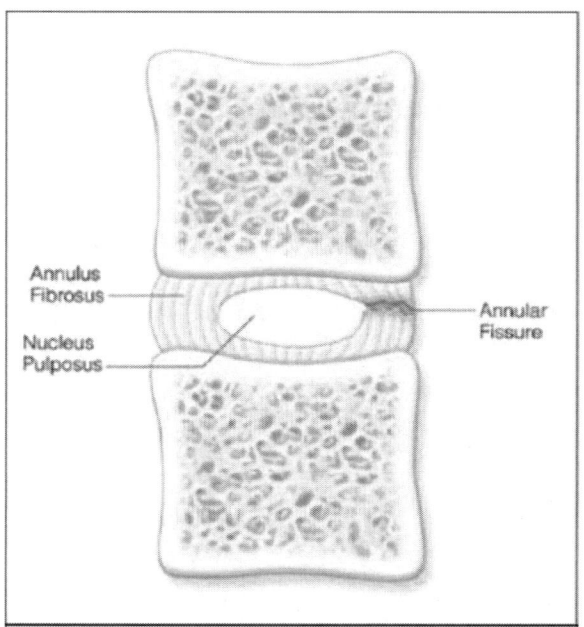

Figure 2. Sagittal and axial schematics of the intervertebral discs depicting a torn annulus fibrosis and herniated nucleus pulposus (Navani et al. 2019).

Vertebral facet joint PRP injections have shown some efficacy for pain. In comparison to corticosteroid injections, PRP injections appear to have delayed onset but longer lasting effects for symptomatic improvement in pain (Akeda et al. 2019). Similar to intradiscal PRP injections, the growth factor-rich supplementation through PRP into the facet joint is hypothesized to decrease the inflammatory profile of the arthritic and inflamed joint and thereby reducing pain (J. Wu et al. 2017).

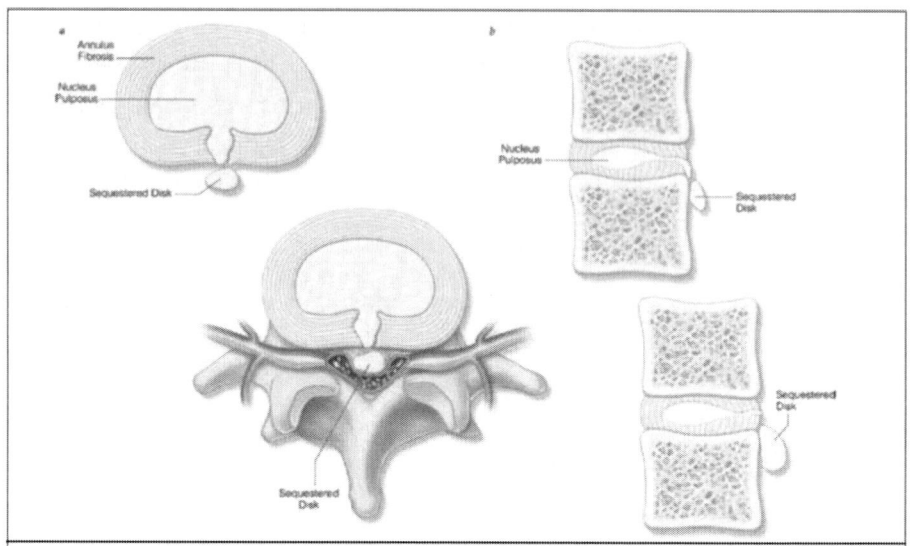

Figure 3. Sagittal and axial schematics of the intervertebral discs depicting a torn annulus fibrosis and herniated nucleus pulposus (Navani et al. 2019).

Bony Regeneration

Bone regeneration is critical for fracture healing and of importance in spine surgery in the setting of bony fusion. *In vitro* studies have demonstrated increased osteogenesis and osteoblast activation by PRP and suggested increased differentiation of human mesenchymal stem cells into osteogenic derivatives (Salamanna et al. 2015). Studies investigating PRP in spine have demonstrated PRP accelerated bony union and reduced time to union *in vivo* in rats and humans. Furthermore, the application of PRP in osteoporosis *in vivo* has demonstrated increased rate of bone healing and improved bone quality, up to limited concentrations as excessively concentrated PRP inhibits complete bone healing (Kinoshita et al. 2020).

POTENTIAL CONTRAINDICTIONS/LIMITATIONS

Limitations of PRP

The primary limitation of PRP in orthopaedics is limited by the paucity of high-level evidence to support broadened usage of PRP in spine surgery. PRP may provide some benefit knee osteoarthritis, however there is inconsistent or minimal benefit of PRP in rotator cuff repairs, patellar tendonopathy, ACL reconstruction, Achilles tendonopathies (Hussain, Johal, and Bhandari 2017).

Potential Contraindications

Unlike exogenous preparations of growth factors, PRP is endogenously derived and therefore a severe immunologic reaction is effectively eliminated. Current contraindications to PRP include infection, thrombocytopenia, systemic steroid use, bone marrow pathology, and therapeutic anticoagulation (Yaari, Dolev, and Haviv 2019). A relative contraindication to PRP is concomitant NSAID use and functional inhibition of platelet activation and aggregation.

Future Directions

In vitro and *in vivo* studies suggest potential for PRP to induce healing and reduce pain through indirect inoculation of growth factors. PRP is a relatively understudied therapeutic in spine surgery and represents an area where high level, randomized, prospective clinical trials are needed to further characterize the efficacy as a therapeutic. At the present, the paucity of both prospective and retrospective clinical trials limits the ability to perform high-quality meta-analysis. Another consideration for future study is assessment of cost effectiveness of PRP compared to current treatments, specifically in spinal fusions in comparison to bone morphogenic protein (BMP).

STEM CELLS

Introduction

Stem cells have grown popular as a cutting-edge treatment for a myriad of spine pathologies. Their robust plasticity and differentiability support their standing as an attractive therapeutic solution for challenging spine conditions. Research efforts are dedicated to comprehending their biology as we strive to understand their therapeutic value in the clinical context. This section aims to discuss stem cell mechanism of action, evaluate the existing evidence regarding stem cell efficacy, current limitations, and future areas of interest.

Biology and Mechanism of Action

Stem cells are undifferentiated cellular precursors with the ability to proliferate and differentiate into various cells and tissues. Each cell's capacity to regenerate depends upon its existing degree of maturation. Understanding stem cell biologic potential allows for appropriate selection and targeted therapy of spinal pathologies (Figure 1). For example, totipotent stem cells – extracted from the developing blastocyst – demonstrate the highest degree of potency and self-renewal which provides greater plasticity. In contrast, unipotent cells – such as osteoblasts – are designed to differentiate into a single cell type (Kolios and Moodley 2012; Ali et al. 2016; Daley 2015).

However, multipotent cells – specifically mesenchymal stem cells (MSC) – are the most commonly used subtype for the treatment of musculoskeletal pathologies because they are the precursors for osteoblasts, chondroblasts, adipocytes, and other cell types (Figure 1). RUNX2 and

SOX9 plays a pivotal role in the differentiation and maturation of MSCs into osteocytes and chondrocytes (Goldring 2012; Komori 2019). MSCs are routinely harvested from bone marrow, synovial tissue, umbilical cord, adipose tissue, peripheral blood, etc. (Sakaguchi et al. 2005; Vadalà et al. 2016; Mushahary et al. 2018; R. H. Lee et al. 2004; Chamberlain et al. 2007). Unfortunately, their regenerative potentials are not equal as MSC isolated from synovial tissue show greater chondrogenic potency (Ando et al. 2014). Interestingly, MSCs primarily function by creating a nutrient-rich environment that facilitates bone healing, not through direct osteoblastic formation. Their regenerative capacity stems from their immunosuppressive or proinflammatory phenotypes which are strongly driven by unique toll-like receptors (TLR) (Oryan et al. 2017; Raicevic et al. 2010; Mo et al. 2008). TLR3 induces immunosuppressive properties which inhibit osteoblastic differentiation.

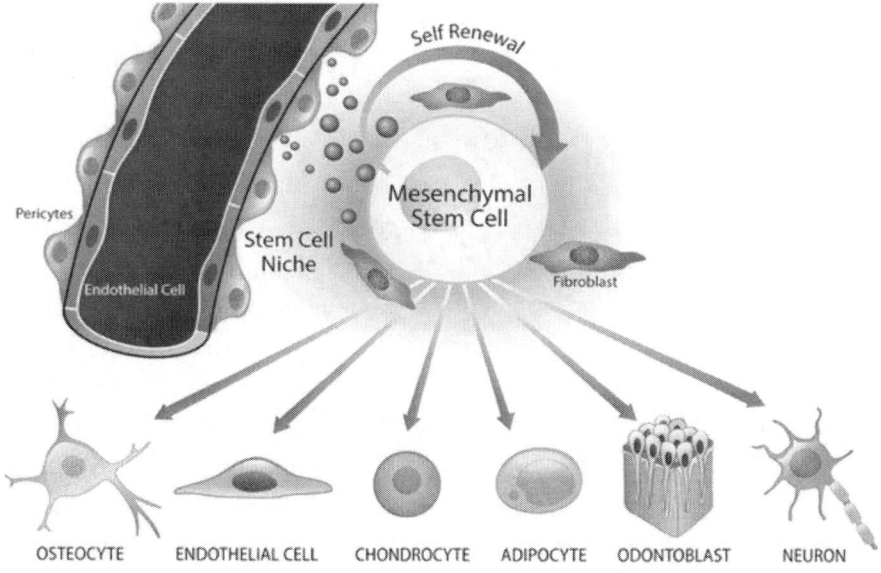

Figure 4. MSC Differentiation. Osteocytes, chondrocytes, and adipocytes are among the different cell types derived from MSCs (Oh and Nör 2015).

In contrast, TL4 stimulates proinflammatory phenotype expression which promotes development of osteoblasts. While MSC differentiation involves a complex interplay between multiple TLRs, TLR3/TLR4 are the primary drivers of differentiation and migration to the target site (Waterman et al. 2010).

Stem Cells in Orthopaedic Surgery

Stem cells have demonstrated a wide range of efficacy in the treatment of musculoskeletal pathologies. Within the field of joint reconstructive surgery, MSCs have been targeted for cartilage regeneration and treatment of osteoarthritis with several *in vitro and in vivo* demonstrating cartilage reconstruction (Diekman et al. 2010; Fong et al. 2012; J. C. Lee et al. 2012; Al Faqeh et al. 2012). Subsequent improvements in functional outcomes and pain scores were reported as well. However, evidence supporting their ability to modify disease course is equivocal. Failure to mimic the unique exact structure and integrity mitigates their effectiveness in altering disease course. Furthermore, MSC do not reliably reverse existing osteophytic changes or peri-articular osseous degeneration – known culprits of joint pain - within the hip or knee (Davatchi et al. 2011).

MSC treatment for ligamentous, tendon, and meniscal injuries has garnered interest in orthopaedic sports surgery. Investigations have shown encouraging results as promising alternatives and adjuvants to conventional therapy. Rotator cuff tendon integrity was evaluated in fourteen patients after delivery of iliac-acquired bone marrow stem cells. At twelve months, tendon integrity was confirmed to be intact by MRI in all patients (Gomes et al. 2012). MSC have also been studied in the context of ACL reconstruction, a common procedure performed by orthopaedic sports surgeons. At one year, knee function and graft incorporation were improved, but these findings did not prove to be statistically significant (Alentorn-Geli et al. 2019). However, a biomechanical study showed tendon pullout resistance was increased after adipose-derived stem cells were administered (X. Zhang et al. 2016). Despite these pronounced results, further Level I evidence is needed to validate their clinical use.

Current Spine Treatments: A Review of the Literature

Intervertebral Disc Degeneration (IDD)

IDD imposes a tremendous burden on spine practices throughout the U.S. With nearly 80% of adults endorsing back-pain related symptoms at some point in their life and a growing geriatric population, targeted degenerative disc therapies are receiving significant attention (Macfarlane et al. 1999). Degenerative changes in the nucleus pulposis coupled with poor chondrocyte plasticity are well-studied and the target of novel stem cell therapies. Degenerating discs experience elevated levels of IL-1, TNF-a, and other local inflammatory cytokines that induce expression of matrix metalloproteinases and disintegrin (Vergroesen et al. 2015). These proteolytic enzymes disrupt the native disc extracellular matrix thus compromising disc integrity and height. Furthermore, the type II collagen and proteoglycan-rich environment is replaced by type I collagen which increases shear forces across the disc (Antoniou et al. 1996). In response, vertebral endplate chondrocytes upregulate nitric oxide production which stimulates cartilage and intervertebral disc apoptosis (Smith, Carter, and Schurman 2004; Hsieh et al. 2004; Liu et al. 2001). Recognizing how MSCs can mitigate and/or reverse the disease process underlying disc degeneration has led to important advances in IDD treatment.

Stem cell treatment is driven by its ability to appropriately differentiate in response to its surrounding environment. Richardson et al. designed a co-culture experiment where MSC differentiation was evaluated when placed in direct contact with the nucleus pulposis. MSC differentiation and extracellular regeneration was elicited after seven days of contact with SOX9. Type II collagen, aggrecan, and mRNA expression was markedly higher in the co-cultured group. In contrast, this upregulation was significantly diminished in the non-contact setting (Richardson et al. 2006).

Several animal trials have exhibited the regenerative capacity of intradiscal MSC injections, specifically by delaying degeneration, increasing type II collagen, and stimulating extracellular matrix growth (Sakai et al. 2003; Y. G. Zhang et al. 2005; Sakai et al. 2006; H. Wang et al. 2014; Hiyama et al. 2008). MSC injections (typically coupled with hyaluronic acid cell carriers) increased disc height and signal on MRI imaging. In one study, 24 adult sheep received either high- or low-dose MSCs at L3-L4 three months after chondroitinase-ABC was injected to artificially generate disc destruction. Restoration to baseline disc height was observed at six months. Histologic examination revealed better overall recovery three months in the high-dose cohort and six months in the low-dose cohort (Ghosh et al. 2012).

In vivo human studies reveal MSC treatment increases functional outcomes and reduces lower back pain. Yoshikawa et al. injected MSCs into the lumbar spine of two geriatric women with radicular pain and lumbar spinal stenosis visualized on MRI. MSCs were isolated from iliac bone marrow and delivered with collagen bone sponges directly into the degenerated disc. At two years, both individuals reported improved Visual Analog Scale (VAS) scores and MRI-confirmed intervertebral disc intensity representing increased fluid (Yoshikawa et al. 2010).

Orozco et al. injected autologous MSCs (AuMSC) into ten patients with persistent lower back pain and IDD at L4-L5 and/or L5-S1. All patients had failed a six-month trial of conservative therapy. Results from the study showed water content was increased in the discs receiving AuMSC injections. Appreciable improvements in pain and disability were noted at three months and ultimately reached 71% of maximum outcomes at the end of the study. It is important to mention that mean age was 35, and the annulus fibrosus at the affected levels were intact in all patients (Orozco et al. 2011).

Allogeneic MSC (AlMSC) have borne promising results in the treatment of lower back pain and improved functional outcomes in patients with IDD. A randomized controlled trial investigated the efficacy of allogeneic bone marrow MSC injections in 24 patients with IDD-associated lumbar back pain. The allogeneic MSC cohort demonstrated lower VAS and Oswestry Disability Index scores at 3 months which was sustained at 6- and 12-month intervals. MRI findings demonstrated greater disc height loss in the control group (0.38mm vs 0.04mm), but these results were not statistically significant (Noriega et al. 2017). AlMSC may also provide a more cost-friendly alternative to AuMSC. In contrast to autologous cells, AlMSC permit single-stage delivery without requiring cell procurement from each individual host.

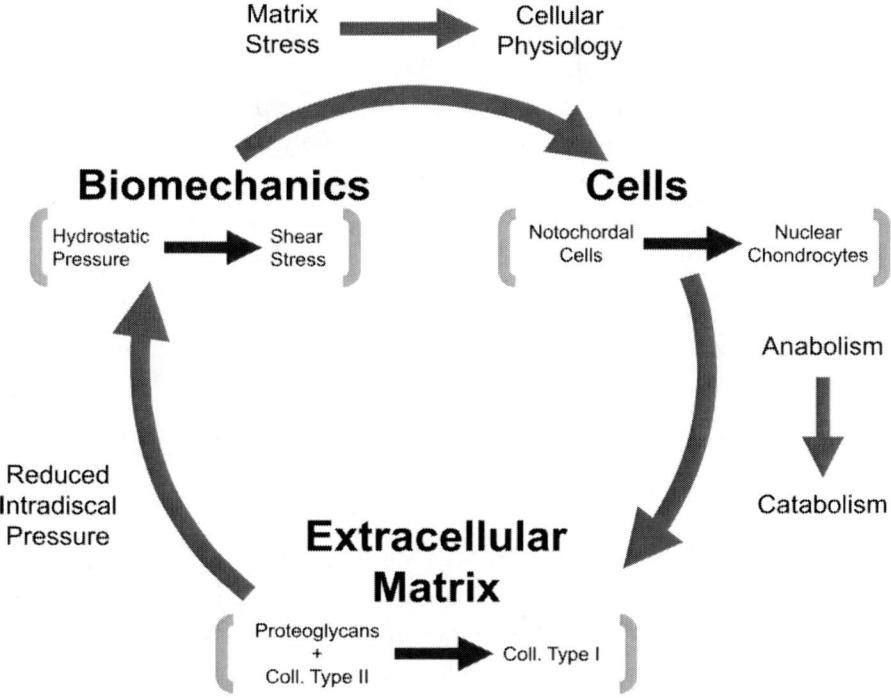

Figure 5. Mechanism and development of IDD (Vergroesen et al. 2015).

Kumar et al. conducted a single-arm phase I clinical trial with ten chronic lower back pain patients to evaluate the safety profile of adipocyte-derived MSC intradiscal injections. Their results showed no adverse events, serious adverse events, or changes in baseline laboratory markers with a single injection throughout the twelve-month period. Intradiscal height was unchanged on plain radiographs, and intradiscal water content was observed in three patients using diffusion-weighted imaging (Kumar et al. 2017).

Spinal Fusion

Single or multiple level vertebral body fusion is a common surgical treatment option for establishing fixation within the spine. Their utility is well-documented within the literature (S. Jain et al. 2016; Mobbs et al. 2015;

Ha et al. 2008; Mobbs et al. 2013; Jiang, Chen, and Jiang 2012). However, these procedures can lead to back pain and instability due to complications associated with nonunion and hardware failure. Augmenting the bone graft with MSCs has shown encouraging findings in these patients.

Gan et al. evaluated 41 patients who underwent posterior spinal fusion (PSF) coupled with porous beta-tricalcium phosphate. Reason for spinal fusion included lumbar instability, spondylosis with stenosis, and thoracolumbar fractures. Concentrated bone marrow aspirate protocols were employed to minimize inconsistencies in MSC yield. At three years, 39/41 patients (95.1%) demonstrated radiographic and computed tomographic evidence of fusion. 21/22 patients (95.5%) undergoing PSF for IDD experienced motor and sensory dexterity improvements from baseline. Worsening of neurologic symptoms in the remaining patients was not observed. MSC donor site morbidity was absent in all patients (Gan et al. 2008).

Taghavi et al. supplemented PSF with bone marrow aspirates containing MSC in eighteen patients. Patients were followed for an average length of 27 months. At the conclusion of the study, successful fusion was observed in all single-level fusions. Nonunions were only observed in the multi-level fusion cohort (7/11 patients). VAS scores at two-year follow-up were significantly higher than preoperatively. Of note, the BMA fusion rates were lower and revision rates were higher as compared to the recombinant human bone morphogenic protein-2 and iliac crest autograft cohorts (Taghavi et al. 2010).

Yousef et al. performed a single-site retrospective study to examine postoperative clinical and radiographic outcomes in 21 patients receiving MSC augment at the time of posterior spinal fusion. Full bilateral fusion was appreciated in all but one patient (unilateral fusion at one level) as confirmed by X-ray and advanced imaging. Only two patients required revision surgery which were performed at four years and five years after the index procedures (Yousef, La Maida, and Misaggi 2017).

Spondyloarthropathies (SA)

Inflammatory spine diseases are a collection of multi-faceted rheumatologic conditions that affect 1.7-2.7 million people in the United States. These diseases include ankylosing spondylitis (AS), psoriatic arthritis, reactive arthritis, arthritis related to inflammatory bowel disease and undifferentiated SA. SA usually presents as a constellation of symptoms including axial inflammation, peripheral arthritis, enthesitis, dactylitis, psoriasis, uveitis and inflammatory bowel disease. Axial skeleton changes are characterized by asymmetrical degenerative joint changes with associated sacroiliitis and spondylitis (Wong 2015; Carli et al. 2019; A. Jones et al. 2018). Contrary to degenerative disc disease, SA is routinely diagnosed in younger populations (usually within the first three decades of life). The wide range of symptoms observed can be attributed to the body's upregulated inflammatory response which alters vertebral bone and joint integrity. While the precise pathophysiology remains controversial, SA is associated with multiple biomarkers. Most prominently, Human Leukocyte Antigen-27 (HLA-27), a major histocompatibility complex, is present in nearly 90% of patients with AS but at a lower percentage in other SA types (van der Linden et al. 1984).

Traditionally, SA treatment has involved a combination of non-steroidal anti-inflammatory drugs, disease-modifying antirheumatic drugs, and corticosteroid injections. These treatment modalities have shown benefit in slowing SA but have long-term implications (Ward et al. 2019; Garcia-Montoya, Gul, and Emery 2018; Braun and Baraliakos 2009). MSC are an evolving therapy with significant clinical promise in SA spinal pathologies.

A clinical trial by Wang et al. aimed to investigate MSC efficacy over a 20-week period in 35 AS patients whom had failed NSAID therapy. AlMSC aspirates were obtained from healthy subjects without any history of AS. The Ankylosing Spondylitis Response Criteria 20 was employed to evaluate clinical symptom changes. Criteria for improvement was reached by 77.4% of subjects by week 4 and was sustained for 7.1 weeks. Total inflammation extent – an evaluation of inflammation measured on MRI – was decreased by approximately 25% at the conclusion of the trial (P. Wang et al. 2014).

Current Limitations and Controversies

Limitations

In the setting of rapid biologic advancement in spine surgery, acknowledging issues with efficacy and safety is crucial. MSC therapy stands as a unique therapeutic option for IDD but is not without limitations. AlMSC demonstrate an acceptable safety profile with few complications documented in spine clinical trials. The reduced major histocompatibility complex I/II expression and innate anti-inflammatory characteristics minimize the host immunologic response after transplantation. However, allogeneic stem cell rejection is not to be overlooked and has been observed in the literature. (Hu et al. 2020; Harding et al. 2019)

Similar to MSCs, hemopoietic stem cells have been suggested as a potential treatment option. However, limited evidence exists to support this notion. A prospective analysis by Hauf et al. investigated how intradiscal HSC injections affect vertebral disc regeneration. Clinical evaluations were performed at 6- and 12-month intervals. No improvement in lower back pain was reported by any patient throughout the duration of the study (Haufe and Mork 2006).

Unfortunately, there is growing evidence that suggests MSC may also have a harmful impact on patients diagnosed with SA. Research shows decreased MSC immune modulating capacity when transplanted into AS patients. This is driven primarily by an increase in the T helper 17/regulatory T-cell ratio in SA-acquired MSC. These changes were not observed in MSC isolated from otherwise healthy patients (P. Wang et al. 2014). In this setting, MSC delivery into the spine may potentiate further osteophyte development in SA patients.

Treatment of large osseous defects with MSCs may be potentially contraindicated. Difficulty establishing a framework to bridge the two fracture ends while allowing growth can impede union. However, the invention of biomaterial carriers – hydrogel, scaffold, etc. – may better facilitate delivery of MSCs and bone growth in these large voids (Oryan et al. 2017; Morishita et al. 2006).

Controversies

Despite tangible benefits within the literature, stem cell therapy remains controversial. Concerns regarding consistency arise due to variations in MSC concentrations during the acquisition process. Aspirate yields varying from 1 in 5,000 to 100,000 cells highlight the importance of protocolized harvesting to minimize dosing variations (Hsu et al. 2012). Furthermore, the cost associated with harvesting is substantial. AlMSCs can mitigate these costs by circumventing the need for autologous MSC harvesting and multi-staged approach as discussed earlier (Malik and Durdy 2015). However, the manufacturing process surrounding AlMSC commercial harvesting remains costly as well (Simaria et al. 2014; Lipsitz et al. 2017). For these reasons, it is imperative that providers engage in open dialogue with each patient regarding the risks, benefits, and alternatives of MSC treatment.

Ethical concerns regarding stem cell therapy present a significant barrier to their implementation. One point of contention is where these grafts are collected. As discussed earlier in this chapter, stem cells encompass a wide gamut of cell progenitors. Much controversy stems from how stem cell harvesting affects the embryo. Embryonic stem cell collection ultimately results in termination of the embryo. MSCs avoid this issue as they are harvested from bone marrow, peripheral blood, and other adult tissue (de Miguel-Beriain 2015). Donor site morbidity may be a sequela, but mortality rate from is not an active concern.

Additionally, certain patient populations exercise their perogative to refuse cellular transfusions, and it is the provider's responsibility to engage in an honest and collaborative discussion regarding stem cells.

Future Directions

An evaluation of the published evidence suggests stem cell therapy may be a beneficial therapeutic modality for IDD treatment, SA, and vertebral interbody fusion, but clinicians are advised to counsel their patients regarding the existing risks and limitations prior to beginning treatment. While stem cells offer tremendous promise, their potential in treating spinal musculoskeletal pathologies is only beginning to be understood. Iatrogenic dural tears, spinal cord injury, and post-operative infection are among the many serious complications associated with open spine procedures. Stem cells afford a less-invasive treatment option that may provide a solution to these operative complications. Additionally, the complex interplay between stem cells and other biologics may alter how physicians and scientists tackle spine pathologies. PRP injections, exosome delivery, and other biologics confer unique opportunities for combination therapy. As we continue to elucidate the utility of stem cells, further investigations into stem cell treatments becomes paramount.

EXOSOMES

Introduction

Cells are known to secrete a variety of vesicles into the extracellular space. The identity of the secreted vesicle and its contents are diverse and depend on many factors. The cell's origin, microenvironment, resting state, level of chemical and physical stress, and the presence of soluble agonists are all factors that can influence a cell's secretome (Vlassov et al. 2012; Tetta et al. 2011). Exosomes are a subclass of secreted extracellular vesicles (EVs) and were first coined by Trams et al. in 1981 while describing secreted vesicles with ectozyme activity (Vlassov et al. 2012). The term exosome as they described it and as we use it is not to be confused with the "exosome" commonly used to describe the mRNA degradosome in eukaryotic cells (Vlassov et al. 2012).

Exosomes have become increasingly attractive as a therapeutic platform due to their size, ability to deliver and exchange intercellular chemical messages, and their role in intracellular communication (Deatheragea and Cooksona 2012). To date, research has found exosomes to be secreted by all cell types in culture, such as epithelial, fibroblast, hematopoietic, immune, placental, tumor, stem, and Schwann cells (Théry, Ostrowski, and Segura 2009; Valenti et al. 2007; Pap et al. 2009; Fevrier et al. 2004; Vlassov et al.

2012). Consistent with this diverse range of cell types, exosomes are also found in urine, breast milk, bronchial lavage fluid, and human blood, suggesting exosome secretion is an important and conserved cellular function (Admyre et al. 2003; Pisitkun, Shen, and Knepper 2004; Caby et al. 2005; Vlassov et al. 2012). Although EVs were originally thought to be inert byproducts of cell damage or plasma membrane turnover, the discovery of EVs, specifically exosomes, as carriers of not only proteins, but genetic information has spurred interest in the potential use of exosomes in diagnostics, therapeutics, regenerative medicine, and in the treatment of chronic diseases such as diabetes mellitus, cancer, and Parkinson's Disease (Siekevitz 1972; Vizoso et al. 2017; Ratajczak et al. 2012; Chang et al. 2018; S. F. Wu et al. 2020; Vlassov et al. 2012; Tetta et al. 2011). In this section of the chapter, we will explore the biogenesis of exosomes, their composition, the potential advantages of exosomes compared to other regenerative techniques, and the experimental evidence that suggests their potential role in the treatment of spinal conditions. We will also discuss current limitations in exosomal research and suggest future applications in order to make the use of exosomes efficacious in a clinical setting.

Exosomes: Definition, Biogenesis, Mechanism of Action

Exosomes are currently identified intracellularly by their unique origin. Exosomes are the only EV known to originate via invagination of endolysosomal vesicles (Yeh Yeo et al. 2013). Upon invagination, exosomes are then stored as intraluminal vesicles (ILVs) within multivesicular bodies (MVBs) of the late endosome, which are regarded as precursors to exosomes (Chung et al. 2020; Simons and Raposo 2009). The biochemical composition of each exosome is dependent on the type of cell and its pathophysiological state (Chung et al. 2020). Once MVBs fuse with the plasma membrane, ILVs are secreted into the extracellular space and become exosomes (Huotari and Helenius 2011; "Aggf1 Attenuates Hepatic Inflammation and Activation of Hepatic Stellate Cells by Repressing Ccl2 Transcription" 2016). Exosomes remain inactive until they reach their target cell (Chung et al. 2020). This endolysosomal derivation restricts the size of exosomes and how much cargo they can hold. When taking into consideration the thickness of the lipid-bilayer, the internal volume of exosomes ranges from 4.2 – 380 yl (10^{-24} l). This permits a carrying capacity to 100 proteins or less, and 10,000 or less nucleic acid nucleotides (Vlassov et al. 2012). Extracellularly, exosomes are differentiated from other EVs by the following parameters: (1) diameters of 30-150nm, (2) flotation density of 1.1-1.18g/ml in sucrose, and (3) the presence of lipid rafts in their lipid-bilayers.

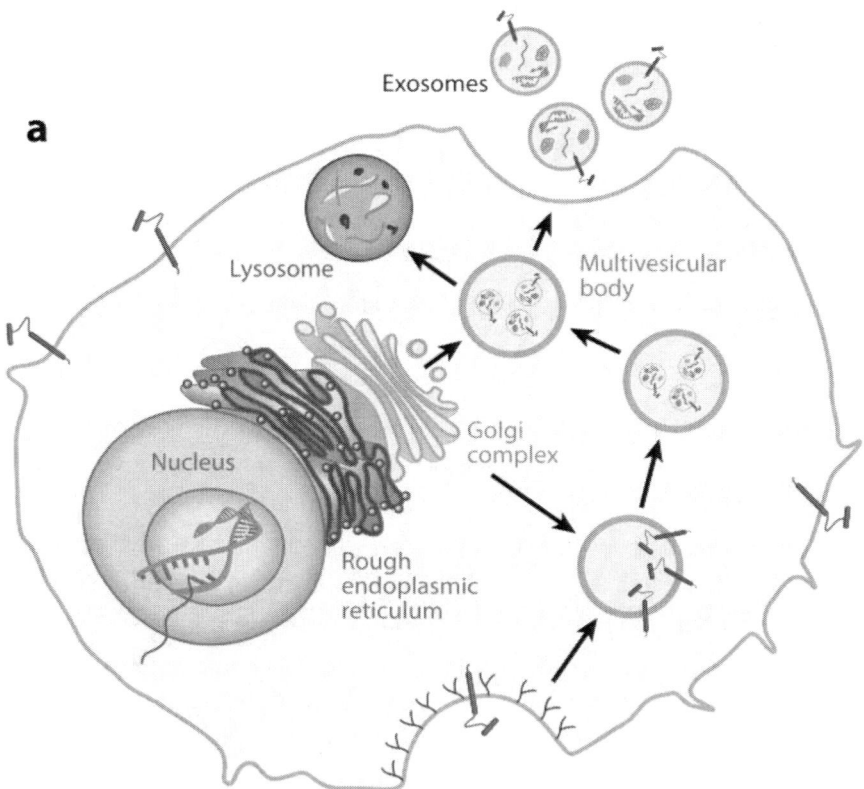

Figure 6. Endolysosomal origin of exosomes via plasma membrane invagination.

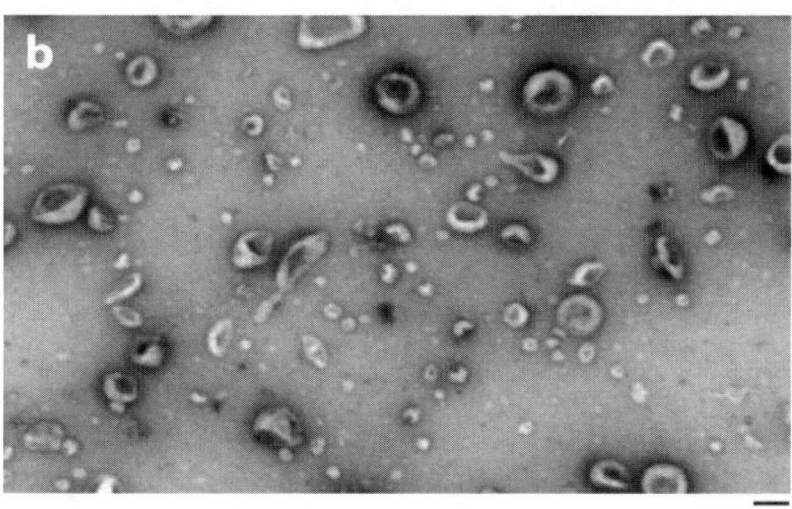

100 nM

Figure 7. Exosome size and structure as seen under electron microscopy (Kourembanas 2015).

Lipid rafts are areas of the membrane involved in the genesis of MVBs and fusion with plasma membranes. Lipid rafts are rich in cholesterol, sphingomyelin, and ceramide (Tanaka et al. 2013; Wubbolts et al. 2003; De Gassart et al. 2003; Chung et al. 2020; Vlassov et al. 2012; Yeh Yeo et al. 2013). Because identification and purification techniques cannot distinguish secreted EVs based on their origin, researchers rely on these characteristics in order to purify their samples. Vlassov et al. reports that the most common method of purification relies on ultracentrifugation of the sample fluid after it has been cleared by a series of lower-speed spins. Pelleting at 100,000-110,000xg, followed by resuspensions and repelleting results in the exosomal sample. The sample can be further purified using sucrose cushions by relying on their aforementioned density to separate the exosomes from any remaining cellular debris (Vlassov et al. 2012).

Along with the characteristics listed above, exosomes from different cellular sources also share a set of protein complexes due to their endosomal origin, such as fusion proteins, membrane transport proteins, and those involved in MVB biogenesis (Vlassov et al. 2012). But besides these similarities, the contents of exosomes are remarkably specific to the identity of the secreting cell (Chung et al. 2020). For example, exosomes secreted by immune cells contain MHC complexes and molecules to induce immune cell proliferation, while exosomes secreted by tumor cells contain factors that inhibit the immune response and enhance tumor progression and metastases (Neviani and Fabbri 2015; "Aggf1 Attenuates Hepatic Inflammation and Activation of Hepatic Stellate Cells by Repressing Ccl2 Transcription" 2016; Yeh Yeo et al. 2013). A database called ExoCarta, an exosome-based community resource, reports greater than 9,000 different proteins and over 6,000 different RNAs (mRNA and miRNA) recovered from exosomal research (Mathivanan and Simpson 2009). This variation in cargo allows for intercellular communication and transfer of genetic information upon fusion with the target cell (Tetta et al. 2011; Vlassov et al. 2012). Their unique composition also provides exosomes with a cell-specific manner to dock and unload their cargo. This unique affinity for their cell target makes exosomes very potent mechanisms to transport proteins, miRNA, and other messenger molecules in the body without being degraded (Burke et al. 2016).

Advantages of Exosome-Based Treatment

Researchers have posited several advantages to using exosomes over other biologic treatments. First, due to their lipid-bilayer and lack of biological markers on the surface of their plasma membrane, exosomes are resistant to degradation. This increases the bioavailability of exosomal cargo and its potential therapeutic effects on target cells when compared to proteinaceous injections or stem cells, which are either quickly degraded or fail to differentiate into the target tissue (Han et al. 2016; Behera and Tyagi 2018; Yeh Yeo et al. 2013). Additionally, exosomes are not "alive," and are therefore easier to handle. This increases their stability and provides the opportunity for storage of exosomes for over two years without loss of function (Vlassov et al. 2012). Exosomes can then be used directly after storage as they are static biochemical entities (Vlassov et al. 2012). Second, many of the therapeutic benefits derived from stem cells has been attributed to their secretion of exosomes. This means exosomes provide a safer alternative to stem cells as they do not carry the risk of disease progression and/or proliferation, while maintaining the beneficial effects (Basu and Ludlow 2016; Han et al. 2016). Third, exosomes can be easily harvested through minimally invasive procedures, such as from bone marrow. This makes them readily available in almost all patients. Also, stem cells have been found to release exosomes in response to distress. Exosomes can therefore be extracted from stem cells under certain conditions in the laboratory, allowing for further exosomal production and analysis of content (Burke et al. 2016; Behera and Tyagi 2018). Lastly, exosomes produced from mesenchymal stem cells (MSCs) or targeted cells (osteocytes, myocytes, chondrocytes, etc.) bypass any ethical concerns that may arise from the use of embryonic stem cells (ESCs) while still eliminating the risk of disease progression and/or proliferation (Yeh Yeo et al. 2013).

Exosomes in Spine Surgery

While exosomal research has spurred in recent decades, its implications in spinal surgery are only in the beginning stages. Here we will discuss results from exosomal studies that address factors that influence the outcomes of spine surgery, such as diabetes mellitus (DM) and osteoporosis, as well as studies that directly deal with orthopedic spinal pathologies, such as intervertebral disc degeneration (IDD) and spinal cord injury (SCI).

Osteoporosis

As the world's population ages and lives longer, osteoporosis is an increasingly prevalent problem worldwide that is caused by negative bone remodeling. Because osteoporosis causes decreased bone density, it is associated with poor outcomes in spinal fusion surgeries due to delayed healing, decreased fusion rates and bone stability (Park and Chung 2011). Due to an increasing life expectancy, the number of patients with osteoporosis will increase as will the need for treatment strategies to affectively address osteoporosis in the setting of spine surgery. Prior treatments options have included anti-absorptive agents that work to increase osteoclast apoptosis, low and infrequent doses of recombinant human PTH that works to increase bone formation, anabolic agents such as bone morphogenic protein (BMP), and implant-based strategies that work to decrease hardware failure (Park and Chung 2011). Emerging research has focused on exosomes and their influence on osteoporosis and other bone disorders.

In a review on the mediators of bone disease, Behera et al. reported osteoblast-derived exosomes activated osteogenesis and bone remodeling through specific signaling molecules while inhibiting osteoclastogenesis. Thus, providing evidence for increased bone formation. MSC-derived exosomes were also found increase formation of blood vessels (angiogenesis) (Behera and Tyagi 2018). Increased angiogenesis is important for bone development, modeling, and growth because it allows for increased delivery of oxygen and nutrients. Adjuvant treatment with osteoblast-derived and MSC-derived exosomes could serve as a viable treatment option for addressing osteoporosis perioperatively and improving outcomes in patients who undergo spinal surgery.

Diabetes Mellitus

Diabetes Type II is another chronic condition that is increasing in prevalence worldwide with increasing rates of obesity and metabolic syndrome. Therefore, more patients with diabetes will be treated and likely undergoing surgery for spinal conditions. While many of the complications associated with DM do not directly influence the musculoskeletal system, the indirect effects can be significant (Wukich 2015). For example, studies have shown poorer outcomes for diabetic patients who undergo spine surgery, such as lower pain improvements, a higher incidence of postoperative complications (incision infection, lower fusion rates, increased bleeding, longer hospital stays, etc.), and poorer return of neurologic function (Satake et al. 2013; Takahashi et al. 2013; Pull Ter Gunne et al. 2012; Wukich 2015). Possible explanations for the poor osteogenic and neurologic outcomes include nerve damage and impaired osteoblast and osteoclast activity in patients with DM (Inaba et al. 1995; Kasahara et al. 2010; K. B. Jones et al. 2005; Inaba et al. 1999; Khazai, Beck, and Umpierrez 2009; Massé et al. 2010; Freedman et al. 2011). Thus, exosomes offer a promising treatment options for patients with DM undergoing spinal surgery.

As stated previously, osteoblast-derived exosomes activated osteogenesis and bone remodeling, while MSC-derived exosomes increased angiogenesis. Both are important processes in ensuring arthrodesis and could provide more positive outcomes for patients with DM. Further, exosomes from human induced pluripotent stem cells-derived MSCs have been shown to accelerate wound healing via enhanced collagen synthesis and angiogenesis, which could lower the risk for postoperative infection and potentially decrease length of stay in hospitals (J. Zhang et al. 2015). Lastly, a recent study by B. Fan et al. found that injecting MSC-derived exosomes into mice with DM ameliorated peripheral neuropathy, which could dampen the neurologic effects of DM and improve patient pain scores (Fan et al. 2020). These results from this study and the studies on wound healing and osteogenesis provide promising treatment options to reduce or eliminate the risks associated with spine surgery for patients with DM.

Intervertebral Disc Degeneration (IDD)

IDD is one of the most common causes of low back pain and affects millions of people worldwide, and effects, as many as 97% of people over the age of 50 (Borenstein 2013; Murray et al. 2013; DePalma, Ketchum, and Saullo 2011; D. Chou et al. 2011; Ashton-Miller, Schmatz, and Schultz 1988). Intervertebral discs (IVDs) consist of the fibrous annulus fibrosus which surrounds the nucleus pulposus cells (NPCs) and cartilage on the superior and inferior end-plates of the vertebral bodies (Humzah and Soames 1988; Cloyd et al. 2007). During degeneration, there is increased NPC apoptosis, extracellular matrix destruction, and accumulation of inflammatory factors, which results in poor mechanics and low back pain (Priyadarshani, Li, and Yao 2016). Initially, IDD is conservatively treated with a short period of rest, physical therapy, and pain management (Di Martino et al. 2005; van Tulder, Koes, and Bouter 1997; Waddell 1987; R. Chou et al. 2009; Fritzell et al. 2001). If symptoms fail to improve, the use of surgical intervention may be required in some cases (Di Martino et al.

2005; van Tulder, Koes, and Bouter 1997; Waddell 1987; R. Chou et al. 2009; Fritzell et al. 2001). But because surgical intervention is not always necessary or feasible, there is a need for a long-term conservative treatment option to alleviate low back pain in patients with IDD. Recent studies have shown exosomes as a possible treatment option to slow or reverse the progression of IDD.

A study by C. Xia et al. concluded that MSC-derived exosomes were able to ameliorate IDD through anti-inflammatory and anti-oxidant pathways. Prior studies have concluded that specific cytokines are involved as effectors of IDD and activators of other catabolic processes of IDD (Risbud and Shapiro 2014; Freemont 2009; Tian et al. 2013). Treatment of degenerated discs with MSC-derived exosomes showed attenuated NPC apoptosis when NPCs were treated with an oxidative species. (Xia et al. 2019) Reactive oxygen species (ROS) have been associated with the pathomechanism of IDD due to their role in disrupting mitochondrial function, which has a negative impact on cell homeostasis and increases cell death (Feng et al. 2017; B. Zhang et al. 2017). MSC-derived exosomes were also shown to reduce inflammatory-marker expression, decrease matrix degradation in NP cells, and attenuate mitochondrial dysfunction through replenishment of mitochondrial-related proteins (Xia et al. 2019). Most importantly, MSC-derived exosomes were shown to slow the progression of IDD *in vivo* and delay matrix degradation during the progression of IDD *in vivo* when compared to subjects not treated with MSC-derived exosomes (Xia et al. 2019).

Another study conducted by K. Lu et al. investigated the role of both MSC and NPC-derived exosomes in the treatment of IDD. They found that both MSCs and NPCs secreted exosomes. Exosomes from both sources also underwent uptake by NPCs. Further, NPC-derived exosomes were shown to promote MSC migration and MSC differentiation into NP-like cells (Lu et al. 2017). This finding could provide opportunities for adjuvant treatment with MSCs and exosomes from the diseased tissue and reduce the probability of unwanted MSC proliferation. Lastly, MSC-derived exosomes were shown to increase NPC proliferation and improve extracellular matrix health. While the exact mechanism of IDD is still unclear, the findings listed above provide good starting points for potential therapy.

Cartilaginous tissues are historically difficult to treat due to their avascular nature. Most of the IVD relies on diffusion of nutrients from the vertebral bodies (Kandel, Roberts, and Urban 2008). This makes IVDs vulnerable to loss of a nutrient supply, which has been thought to be a major cause of cell death and disc degeneration (Urban, Smith, and Fairbank 2004). Treatment of the vertebral body with angiogenic exosomes could increase nutrient supply to IVDs and slow progression IDD. Treatment with MSC and NPC-derived exosomes could follow treatment of angiogenic exosomes to slow the progression of IDD even further.

Spinal Cord Injury (SCI)

While SCI is less common than degenerative spinal pathologies, many patients may present with conditions that have caused long-term and potentially permanent neurological damage. Although the specific mechanism of SCI is not clear, it has been associated with neuronal cell apoptosis and activation of inflammatory pathways (Huang et al. 2017). Several studies have shown neuronal cell and MSC-derived exosomes to attenuate neuronal cell apoptosis, inflammation, induce angiogenesis, and promote recovery following SCI (Al-Nedawi et al. 2009; Cai et al. 2012; Zhuang et al. 2012; Kim et al. 2018; Li et al. 2018). These findings suggest neurological treatment with exosomes could decrease damage and accelerate neurologic recovery caused by various spinal pathologies.

Additional Comments

It is also important to mention that MSC-derived exosomes have also been implicated in skeletal muscle regeneration by promoting myogenesis and angiogenesis. Although the mechanism is not known, exosomes could also be used as a therapeutic tool following invasive surgeries to aid in the healing process as many patients experience severe postoperative surgical pain (Naguibneva et al. 2006; Behera and Tyagi 2018).

Last Comments

Lastly, while we mentioned exosomes for use in patients with osteoporosis, DM, IDD, and SCI, it is inherent in the presented research that many of these interventions could also be used with patients who do not present with these diagnoses. The exciting implications in exosomal research lies in their potential to improve patient outcomes and lessen pre- and post-operative complications for all patients. For example, increased bone formation and modeling is sought for any patient undergoing spinal fusion, not just those with chronic diseases; decreased risk of infection via rapid wound healing is advantageous for all patients, not just those with DM.

Potential Contraindications and Limitations

All available research supports the use of exosomes in diagnostics, therapeutics, regenerative medicine, and in the treatment of chronic diseases. However, there are still issues that need to be addressed before exosomes can be used in a clinical setting. First, there are limitations in the manufacturing and production of exosomes. Laboratory yield of exosomes is typically less than 1μg per 1mL of culture medium, where the useful dose is typically 10-100 μg per mouse in recent studies (Yamashita, Takahashi, and Takakura 2018; Lv et al. 2018; Charoenviriyakul et al. 2017; Yamashita et al. 2016; Willis, Kourembanas, and Mitsialis 2017). Thus a means to produce larger amounts of exosomes is required. Additionally, there is a lack of defining markers when identifying exosomes. Current techniques rely on size or the presence of specific protein complexes, but these methods are often cumbersome or too generic. Thus, there is a need for an unambiguous assay to accurately identify and collect exosomes (Yeh Yeo et al. 2013). Secondly, while there is evidence of specific proteins, nucleic acids, and other biochemical factors involved in exosome pathology, no clear mechanism has been deduced (Chung et al. 2020). Further, exosomes have been implicated in the progression of cancer and degenerative and infectious diseases (Yeh Yeo et al. 2013). When considered together, these factors enhance the need to validate the mechanism of exosomal function if they are to proceed to clinical application.

Future Directions

Ideally, future exosome research will discover the pathogenesis of exosome action in treatment of chronic diseases. Once these mechanisms have been deduced, there is a need for extensive clinical trials to address the potential use of exosomes in spine-specific pathologies, such as surgical outcomes in osteoporotic or diabetic patients, the incidence of postoperative infections, and fusion rates in non-diseased patients to examine the efficacy of in-vivo exosome therapy. This will allow for the creation of novel exosomes specific to the disorder being addressed, which would result in improved clinical outcomes (Behera and Tyagi 2018). Much research will need to be done given the diverse and widespread influence of exosomes, but they remain a promising therapy for a variety of diseases and offer improved outcomes in the treatment of common spinal pathologies.

REFERENCES

Admyre, Charlotte, Grunewald, J., Thyberg, J., Bripenäck, S., Tornling, G., Eklund, A., Scheynius, A. & Gabrielsson, S. (2003). "Exosomes with Major Histocompatibility Complex Class II and Co-Stimulatory Molecules Are Present in Human BAL Fluid." *European Respiratory Journal*. https://doi.org/10.1183/09031936.03.00041703.

"Aggf1 Attenuates Hepatic Inflammation and Activation of Hepatic Stellate Cells by Repressing Ccl2 Transcription." 2016. *Journal of Biomedical Research*. https://doi.org/10.7555/jbr.31.20160046.

Akeda, K., Yamada, J, Linn, E. T., Sudo, A. & Masuda, K. (2019). "Platelet-Rich Plasma in the Management of Chronic Low Back Pain: A Critical Review." *J Pain Res*, 12, 753–67. https://doi.org/10.2147/JPR.S153085.

Al-Nedawi, Khalid, Brian Meehan, Robert S. Kerbel, Anthony C. Allison. & Anusz Rak. (2009). "Endothelial Expression of Autocrine VEGF upon the Uptake of Tumor-Derived Microvesicles Containing Oncogenic EGFR." *Proceedings of the National Academy of Sciences of the United States of America.* https://doi.org/10.1073/pnas.0804543106.

Alentorn-Geli, Eduard, Roberto Seijas, Adrián Martínez-De la Torre, Xavier Cuscó, Gilbert Steinbacher, Pedro Álvarez-Díaz, David Barastegui., et al. (2019). "Effects of Autologous Adipose-Derived Regenerative Stem Cells Administered at the Time of Anterior Cruciate Ligament Reconstruction on Knee Function and Graft Healing." *Journal of Orthopaedic Surgery.* https://doi.org/10.1177/ 2309499019867580.

Ali, F., Taresh, S., Al-Nuzaily, M., Mok, P. L., Ismail, A. & Ahmad, S. (2016). "Stem Cells Differentiation and Probing Their Therapeutic Applications in Hematological Disorders: A Critical Review." *European Review for Medical and Pharmacological Sciences.*

Ando, Wataru, Josh J. Kutcher, Roman Krawetz, Arindom Sen, Norimasa Nakamura, Cyril B. Frank. & David A. Hart. (2014). "Clonal Analysis of Synovial Fluid Stem Cells to Characterize and Identify Stable Mesenchymal Stromal Cell/Mesenchymal Progenitor Cell Phenotypes in a Porcine Model: A Cell Source with Enhanced Commitment to the Chondrogenic Lineage." *Cytotherapy.* https://doi.org/10.1016/j.jcyt.2013.12.003.

Antoniou, John, Thomas Steffen, Fred Nelson, Neil Winterbottom, Anthony P. Hollander, Robin A. Poole, Max Aebi. & Mauro Alini. (1996). "The Human Lumbar Intervertebral Disc: Evidence for Changes in the Biosynthesis and Denaturation of the Extracellular Matrix with Growth, Maturation, Ageing, and Degeneration." *Journal of Clinical Investigation.* https://doi.org/10.1172/JCI118884.

Ashton-Miller, James A., Schmatz, C. & Schultz, A. B. (1988). "Lumbar Disc Degeneration: Correlation with Age, Sex, and Spine Level in 600 Autopsy Specimens." *Spine.* https://doi.org/10.1097/00007632-198802000-00008.

Baig, M. Z., Abdullah, U. E. H., Muhammad, A., Aziz, A., Syed, M. J. & Darbar, A. (2020). "Use of Platelet-Rich Plasma in Treating Low Back Pain: A Review of the Current Literature." *Asian Spine J.* https://doi.org/10.31616/asj.2019.0161.

Basu, Joydeep. & John W. Ludlow. (2016). "Exosomes for Repair, Regeneration and Rejuvenation." *Expert Opinion on Biological Therapy.* https://doi.org/10.1517/14712598.2016.1131976.

Behera, Jyotirmaya. & Neetu Tyagi. (2018). "Exosomes: Mediators of Bone Diseases, Protection, and Therapeutics Potential." *Oncoscience.* https://doi.org/10.18632/oncoscience.421.

Borenstein, David. (2013). "Mechanical Low Back Pain - A Rheumatologist's View." *Nature Reviews Rheumatology.* https://doi.org/10.1038/nrrheum.2013.133.

Braun, Juergen. & Xenofon Baraliakos. (2009). "Treatment of Ankylosing Spondylitis and Other Spondyloarthritides." *Current Opinion in Rheumatology.* https://doi.org/10.1097/BOR.0b013e32832c6674.

Burke, John, Ravindra Kolhe, Monte Hunter, Carlos Isales, Mark Hamrick. & Sadanand Fulzele. (2016). "Stem Cell-Derived Exosomes: A Potential Alternative Therapeutic Agent in Orthopaedics." *Stem Cells International.* https://doi.org/10.1155/2016/5802529.

Caby, Marie Pierre, Danielle Lankar, Claude Vincendeau-Scherrer, Graça Raposo. & Christian Bonnerot. (2005). "Exosomal-like Vesicles Are Present in Human Blood Plasma." *International Immunology.* https://doi.org/10.1093/intimm/dxh267.

Cai, Zhijian, Fei Yang, Lei Yu, Zhou Yu, Lingling Jiang, Qingqing Wang, Yunshan Yang, Lie Wang, Xuetao Cao. & Jianli Wang. (2012). "Activated T Cell Exosomes Promote Tumor Invasion via Fas Signaling Pathway." *The Journal of Immunology.*, https://doi.org/10.4049/jimmunol.1103466.

Carli, Linda, Emanuele Calabresi, Gianmaria Governato. & Juergen Braun. (2019). "One Year in Review 2018: Axial Spondyloarthritis." *Clinical and Experimental Rheumatology.*

Chamberlain, Giselle, James Fox, Brian Ashton. & Jim Middleton. (2007). "Concise Review: Mesenchymal Stem Cells: Their Phenotype,

Differentiation Capacity, Immunological Features, and Potential for Homing." *Stem Cells*. https://doi.org/10.1634/stemcells.2007-0197.

Chang, Yu Hsun, Kung Chi Wu, Horng Jyh Harn, Shinn Zong Lin. & Dah Ching Ding. (2018). "Exosomes and Stem Cells in Degenerative Disease Diagnosis and Therapy." *Cell Transplantation*. https://doi.org/10.1177/0963689717723636.

Charoenviriyakul, Chonlada, Yuki Takahashi, Masaki Morishita, Akihiro Matsumoto, Makiya Nishikawa. & Yoshinobu Takakura. (2017). "Cell Type-Specific and Common Characteristics of Exosomes Derived from Mouse Cell Lines: Yield, Physicochemical Properties, and Pharmacokinetics." *European Journal of Pharmaceutical Sciences*. https://doi.org/10.1016/j.ejps.2016.10.009.

Chou, Dean, Dino Samartzis, Carlo Bellabarba, Alpesh Patel, Keith, D. K., Luk, Jeannette, Schenk Kisser, M. & Andrea C. Skelly. (2011). "Degenerative Magnetic Resonance Imaging Changes in Patients with Chronic Low Back Pain: A Systematic Review." *Spine*. https://doi.org/10.1097/BRS.0b013e31822ef700.

Chou, Roger, Jamie Baisden, Eugene J. Carragee, Daniel K. Resnick, William O. Shaffer. & John D. Loeser. (2009). "Surgery for Low Back Pain: A Review of the Evidence for an American Pain Society Clinical Practice Guideline." *Spine*. https://doi.org/10.1097/ BRS.0b013e3 181a105fc.

Chung, Ill Min, Govindasamy Rajakumar, Baskar Venkidasamy, Umadevi Subramanian. & Muthu Thiruvengadam. (2020). "Exosomes: Current Use and Future Applications." *Clinica Chimica Acta*. https://doi.org/10.1016/j.cca.2019.10.022.

Cloyd, Jordan M., Neil R. Malhotra, Lihui Weng, Weiliam Chen, Robert L. Mauck. & Dawn M. Elliott. (2007). "Material Properties in Unconfined Compression of Human Nucleus Pulposus, Injectable Hyaluronic Acid-Based Hydrogels and Tissue Engineering Scaffolds." *European Spine Journal*. https://doi.org/10.1007/s00586-007-0443-6.

Daley, George Q. (2015). "Stem Cells and the Evolving Notion of Cellular Identity." *Philosophical Transactions of the Royal Society B: Biological Sciences*. https://doi.org/10.1098/rstb.2014.0376.

Davatchi, Fereydoun, Bahar Sadeghi Abdollahi, Mandana Mohyeddin, Farhad Shahram. & Behrooz Nikbin. (2011). "Mesenchymal Stem Cell Therapy for Knee Osteoarthritis. Preliminary Report of Four Patients." *International Journal of Rheumatic Diseases*. https://doi.org/10.1111/j.1756-185X.2011.01599.x.

Deatheragea, Brooke L. & Brad T. Cooksona. (2012). "Membrane Vesicle Release in Bacteria, Eukaryotes, and Archaea: A Conserved yet Underappreciated Aspect of Microbial Life." *Infection and Immunity*. https://doi.org/10.1128/IAI.06014-11.

Delgado, D., Garate, A., Vincent, H., Bilbao, A. M., Patel, R., Fiz, N., Sampson, S. & Sanchez, M. (2019). "Current Concepts in Intraosseous Platelet-Rich Plasma Injections for Knee Osteoarthritis." *J Clin Orthop Trauma*, 10 (1), 36–41. https://doi.org/10.1016/j.jcot.2018.09.017.

DePalma, Michael J., Jessica M. Ketchum. & Thomas Saullo. (2011). "What Is the Source of Chronic Low Back Pain and Does Age Play a Role?" *Pain Medicine*. https://doi.org/10.1111/j.1526-4637.2010.01045.x.

Diekman, Brian O., Christopher R. Rowland, Donald P. Lennon, Arnold I. Caplan. & Farshid Guilak. (2010). "Chondrogenesis of Adult Stem Cells from Adipose Tissue and Bone Marrow: Induction by Growth Factors and Cartilage-Derived Matrix." In *Tissue Engineering - Part A*. https://doi.org/10.1089/ten.tea.2009.0398.

Fan, Baoyan, Chao Li, Alexandra Szalad, Lei Wang, Wanlong Pan, Ruilan Zhang, Michael Chopp, Zheng Gang Zhang. & Xian Shuang Liu. (2020). "Mesenchymal Stromal Cell-Derived Exosomes Ameliorate Peripheral Neuropathy in a Mouse Model of Diabetes." *Diabetologia*. https://doi.org/10.1007/s00125-019-05043-0.

Faqeh, Hamoud Al, Bin Mohamad Yahya Nor Hamdan, Hui Cheng Chen, Bin Saim Aminuddin. & Bt Hj Idrus Ruszymah. (2012). "The Potential of Intra-Articular Injection of Chondrogenic-Induced Bone Marrow Stem Cells to Retard the Progression of Osteoarthritis in a Sheep Model." *Experimental Gerontology*. https://doi.org/10.1016/ j.exger.2012.03.018.

Feng, Chencheng, Minghui Yang, Minghong Lan, Chang Liu, Yang Zhang, Bo Huang, Huan Liu. & Yue Zhou. (2017). "ROS: Crucial

Intermediators in the Pathogenesis of Intervertebral Disc Degeneration." *Oxidative Medicine and Cellular Longevity.* https://doi.org/10.1155/2017/5601593.

Fevrier, Benoit, Didier Vilette, Fabienne Archer, Damarys Loew, Wolfgang Faigle, Michel Vidal, Hubert Laude. & Graça Raposo. (2004). "Cells Release Prions in Association with Exosomes." *Proceedings of the National Academy of Sciences of the United States of America.* https://doi.org/10.1073/pnas.0308413101.

Fong, Chui Yee, Arjunan Subramanian, Kalamegam Gauthaman, Jayarama Venugopal, Arijit Biswas, Seeram Ramakrishna. & Ariff Bongso. (2012). "Human Umbilical Cord Wharton's Jelly Stem Cells Undergo Enhanced Chondrogenic Differentiation When Grown on Nanofibrous Scaffolds and in a Sequential Two-Stage Culture Medium Environment." *Stem Cell Reviews and Reports.* https://doi.org/10.1007/s12015-011-9289-8.

Freedman, Mitchell K., Alan S. Hilibrand, Emily A. Blood, Wenyan Zhao, Todd J. Albert, Alexander R. Vaccaro, Christina V. Oleson, Tamara S. Morgan. & James N. Weinstein. (2011). "The Impact of Diabetes on the Outcomes of Surgical and Nonsurgical Treatment of Patients in the Spine Patient Outcomes Research Trial." *Spine.* https://doi.org/10.1097/BRS.0b013e3181ef9d8c.

Freemont, A. J. (2009). "The Cellular Pathobiology of the Degenerate Intervertebral Disc and Discogenic Back Pain." *Rheumatology.* https://doi.org/10.1093/rheumatology/ken396.

Fritzell, Peter, Olle Hägg, Per Wessberg. & Anders Nordwall. (2001). "2001 Volvo Award Winner in Clinical Studies: Lumbar Fusion versus Nonsurgical Treatment for Chronic Low Back Pain. A Multicenter Randomized Controlled Trial from the Swedish Lumbar Spine Study Group." *Spine.* https://doi.org/10.1097/00007632-200112010-00002.

Gan, Yaokai, Kerong Dai, Pu Zhang, Tingting Tang, Zhenan Zhu. & Jianxi Lu. (2008). "The Clinical Use of Enriched Bone Marrow Stem Cells Combined with Porous Beta-Tricalcium Phosphate in Posterior Spinal Fusion." *Biomaterials.* https://doi.org/10.1016/ j.biomaterials.2008.06.026.

Garcia-Montoya, Leticia, Hanna Gul. & Paul Emery. (2018). "Recent Advances in Ankylosing Spondylitis: Understanding the Disease and Management [Version 1; Peer Review: 2 Approved]." *F1000Research*. https://doi.org/10.12688/F1000RESEARCH.14956.1.

Gassart, Aude De, Charles Géminard, Benoit Février, Graça Raposo. & Michel Vidal. (2003). "Lipid Raft-Associated Protein Sorting in Exosomes." *Blood*. https://doi.org/10.1182/blood-2003-03-0871.

Ghosh, Peter, Robert Moore, Barrie Vernon-Roberts, Tony Goldschlager, Diane Pascoe, Andrew Zannettino, Stan Gronthos. & Silviu Itescu. (2012). "Immunoselected STRO-3+ Mesenchymal Precursor Cells and Restoration of the Extracellular Matrix of Degenerate Intervertebral Discs: Laboratory Investigation." *Journal of Neurosurgery: Spine*. https://doi.org/10.3171/2012.1.SPINE11852.

Goldring, Mary B. (2012). "Chondrogenesis, Chondrocyte Differentiation, and Articular Cartilage Metabolism in Health and Osteoarthritis." *Therapeutic Advances in Musculoskeletal Disease*. https://doi.org/10.1177/1759720X12448454.

Gomes, João L.Ellera, Ricardo Canquerini da Silva, Lúcia M. R. Silla, Marcelo R. Abreu. & Roberto Pellanda. (2012). "Conventional Rotator Cuff Repair Complemented by the Aid of Mononuclear Autologous Stem Cells." *Knee Surgery, Sports Traumatology, Arthroscopy*. https://doi.org/10.1007/s00167-011-1607-9.

Greene, A. C. & Hsu, W. K. (2019). "Orthobiologics in Minimally Invasive Lumbar Fusion." *J Spine Surg*, 5, (Suppl 1), S11–18. https://doi.org/10.21037/jss.2019.04.15.

Ha, Kee Yong, Ki Ho Na, Jae Hyuk Shin. & Ki Won Kim. (2008). "Comparison of Posterolateral Fusion with and without Additional Posterior Lumbar Interbody Fusion for Degenerative Lumbar Spondylolisthesis." *Journal of Spinal Disorders and Techniques*. https://doi.org/10.1097/BSD.0b013e3180eaa202.

Hall, M. P., Band, P. A., Meislin, R. J., Jazrawi, L. M. & Cardone, D. A. (2009). "Platelet-Rich Plasma: Current Concepts and Application in Sports Medicine." *J Am Acad Orthop Surg*, 17 (10), 602–8. https://doi.org/10.5435/00124635-200910000-00002.

Han, Chao, Xuan Sun, Ling Liu, Haiyang Jiang, Yan Shen, Xiaoyun Xu, Jie Li., et al. (2016). "Exosomes and Their Therapeutic Potentials of Stem Cells." *Stem Cells International.* https://doi.org/ 10.1155/2016 /7653489.

Harding, Jeffrey, Kristina Vintersten-Nagy, Maria Shutova, Huijuan Yang, Jean Kit Tang, Mohammad Massumi, Mohammad Izaidfar., et al. (2019). "Induction of Long-Term Allogeneic Cell Acceptance and Formation of Immune Privileged Tissue in Immunocompetent Hosts." *BioRxiv.* https://doi.org/10.1101/716571.

Haufe, Scott M. W. & Anthony R. Mork. (2006). "Intradiscal Injection of Hematopoietic Stem Cells in an Attempt to Rejuvenate the Intervertebral Discs." *Stem Cells and Development.* https://doi.org/ 10.1089/scd.2006.15.136.

Hiyama, Akihiko, Joji Mochida, Toru Iwashina, Hiroko Omi, Takuya Watanabe, Kenji Serigano, Futoshi Tamura. & Daisuke Sakai. (2008). "Transplantation of Mesenchymal Stem Cells in a Canine Disc Degeneration Model." *Journal of Orthopaedic Research.* https://doi.org/10.1002/jor.20584.

Hsieh, Adam H., Walsh, A. J. L., Cheng, L. Y. & Lotz, J. C. (2004). "Apoptosis Corresponds with Disc Strain Environment during Dynamic Compression." In *Transactions of the 50th Annualmeeting of the Orthopaedic Research Society.*

Hsu, Wellington K., Nickoli, M. S., Wang, J. C., Lieberman, J. R., An, H. S., Yoon, S. T., Youssef, J. A., Brodke, D. S. & McCullough, C. M. (2012). "Improving the Clinical Evidence of Bone Graft Substitute Technology in Lumbar Spine Surgery." *Global Spine Journal.* https://doi.org/10.1055/s-0032-1315454.

Hu, X., Deuse, T., Gravina, A., Wang, D., Tediashvili, G., De, C., Thayer, W., et al. (2020). "Hypoimmunogenic Derivatives of Induced Pluripotent Stem Cells Evade Immune Rejection in Fully Immunocompetent Allogeneic Recipients." *The Journal of Heart and Lung Transplantation: The Official Publication of the International Society for Heart Transplantation.* https://doi.org/10.1016/ j.healun.2020.01.749.

Huang, Jiang Hu, Xiao Ming Yin, Yang Xu, Chun Cai Xu, Xi Lin, Fu Biao Ye, Yong Cao. & Fei Yue Lin. (2017). "Systemic Administration of Exosomes Released from Mesenchymal Stromal Cells Attenuates Apoptosis, Inflammation, and Promotes Angiogenesis after Spinal Cord Injury in Rats." *Journal of Neurotrauma*. https://doi.org/10.1089/neu.2017.5063.

Humzah, M. D. & Soames, R. W. (1988). "Human Intervertebral Disc: Structure and Function." *The Anatomical Record*. https://doi.org/10.1002/ar.1092200402.

Huotari, Jatta. & Ari Helenius. (2011). "Endosome Maturation." *EMBO Journal*. https://doi.org/10.1038/emboj.2011.286.

Hussain, N., Johal, H. & Bhandari, M. (2017). "An Evidence-Based Evaluation on the Use of Platelet Rich Plasma in Orthopedics - a Review of the Literature." *SICOT J*, 3, 57. https://doi.org/10.1051/sicotj/2017036.

Inaba, Masaaki, Nishizawa, Y., Mita, K., Kumeda, Y., Emoto, M., Kawagishi, T., Ishimura, E., Nakatsuka, K., Shioi, A. & Morii, H. (1999). "Poor Glycemic Control Impairs the Response of Biochemical Parameters of Bone Formation and Resorption to Exogenous 1,25-Dihydroxyvitamin D3 in Patients with Type 2 Diabetes." *Osteoporosis International*. https://doi.org/10.1007/s001980050180.

Inaba, Masaaki, Makoto Terada, Hidenori Koyama, Osamu Yoshida, Eiji Ishimura, Takahiko Kawagishi, Yasuhisa Okuno, Yoshiki Nishizawa, Hirotoshi Morii. & Shuzo Otani. (1995). "Influence of High Glucose on 1,25-dihydroxyvitamin D3-induced Effect on Human Osteoblast-like MG63 Cells." *Journal of Bone and Mineral Research*. https://doi.org/10.1002/jbmr.5650100709.

Jain, A., Yeramaneni, S., Kebaish, K. M., Raad, M., Gum, J. L., Klineberg, E. O., Hassanzadeh, H., et al. (2020). "Cost-Utility Analysis of RhBMP-2 Use in Adult Spinal Deformity Surgery." *Spine (Phila Pa 1976)*. https://doi.org/10.1097/BRS.0000000000003442.

Jain, Sukrit, Adam E. M. Eltorai, Roy Ruttiman. & Alan H. Daniels. (2016). "Advances in Spinal Interbody Cages." *Orthopaedic Surgery*. https://doi.org/10.1111/os.12264.

Jiang, Sheng Dan, Jiang Wei Chen. & Lei Sheng Jiang. (2012). "Which Procedure Is Better for Lumbar Interbody Fusion: Anterior Lumbar Interbody Fusion or Transforaminal Lumbar Interbody Fusion?" *Archives of Orthopaedic and Trauma Surgery*. https://doi.org/10.1007/s00402-012-1546-z.

Jones, Alexis, Coziana Ciurtin, Mediola Ismajli, Maria Leandro, Raj Sengupta. & Pedro M. Machado. (2018). "Biologics for Treating Axial Spondyloarthritis." *Expert Opinion on Biological Therapy*. https://doi.org/10.1080/14712598.2018.1468884.

Jones, Kevin B., Maiers-Yelden, K. A., Marsh, J. L., Zimmerman, M. B., Estin, M. & Saltzman, C. L. (2005). "Ankle Fractures in Patients with Diabetes Mellitus." *Journal of Bone and Joint Surgery - Series B*. https://doi.org/10.1302/0301-620X.87B4.15724.

Kandel, Rita, Sally Roberts. & Jill P.G. Urban. (2008). "Tissue Engineering and the Intervertebral Disc: The Challenges." In *European Spine Journal*. https://doi.org/10.1007/s00586-008-0746-2.

Kasahara, Toshiyuki, Sinji Imai, Hideto Kojima, Miwako Katagi, Hiroshi Kimura, Lawrence Chan. & Yoshitaka Matsusue. (2010). "Malfunction of Bone Marrow-Derived Osteoclasts and the Delay of Bone Fracture Healing in Diabetic Mice." *Bone*. https://doi.org/10.1016/j.bone.2010.06.014.

Kenmochi, M. (2020). "Clinical Outcomes Following Injections of Leukocyte-Rich Platelet-Rich Plasma in Osteoarthritis Patients." *J Orthop*, *18*, 143–49. https://doi.org/10.1016/j.jor.2019.11.041.

Khazai, Natasha B., George R. Beck. & Guillermo E. Umpierrez. (2009). "Diabetes and Fractures: An Overshadowed Association." *Current Opinion in Endocrinology, Diabetes and Obesity*. https://doi.org/10.1097/MED.0b013e328331c7eb.

Kim, Han Young, Hemant Kumar, Min Jae Jo, Jonghoon Kim, Jeong Kee Yoon, Ju Ro Lee, Mikyung Kang., et al. (2018). "Therapeutic Efficacy-Potentiated and Diseased Organ-Targeting Nanovesicles Derived from Mesenchymal Stem Cells for Spinal Cord Injury Treatment." *Nano Letters*. https://doi.org/10.1021/acs.nanolett.8b01816.

Kinoshita, H., Orita, S., Inage, K., Fujimoto, K., Shiga, Y., Abe, K., Inoue, M., et al. (2020). "Freeze-Dried Platelet-Rich Plasma Induces Osteoblast Proliferation via Platelet-Derived Growth Factor Receptor-Mediated Signal Transduction." *Asian Spine J*, *14* (1), 1–8. https://doi.org/10.31616/asj.2019.0048.

Kolios, George. & Yuben Moodley. (2012). "Introduction to Stem Cells and Regenerative Medicine." *Respiration*. https://doi.org/10.1159/000345615.

Komori, Toshihisa. (2019). "Regulation of Proliferation, Differentiation and Functions of Osteoblasts by Runx2." *International Journal of Molecular Sciences*. https://doi.org/10.3390/ijms20071694.

Kourembanas, Stella. (2015). "Exosomes: Vehicles of Intercellular Signaling, Biomarkers, and Vectors of Cell Therapy." *Annual Review of Physiology*, 13–27.

Kumar, Hemant, Doo Hoe Ha, Eun Jong Lee, Jun Hee Park, Jeong Hyun Shim, Tae Keun Ahn, Kyoung Tae Kim., et al. (2017). "Safety and Tolerability of Intradiscal Implantation of Combined Autologous Adipose-Derived Mesenchymal Stem Cells and Hyaluronic Acid in Patients with Chronic Discogenic Low Back Pain: 1-Year Follow-up of a Phase i Study." *Stem Cell Research and Therapy*. https://doi.org/10.1186/s13287-017-0710-3.

Lee, Jae Chul, Sang Young Lee, Hyun Jin Min, Sun Ae Han, Jak Jang, Sahnghoon Lee, Sang Cheol Seong. & Myung Chul Lee. (2012). "Synovium-Derived Mesenchymal Stem Cells Encapsulated in a Novel Injectable Gel Can Repair Osteochondral Defects in a Rabbit Model." *Tissue Engineering - Part A*. https://doi.org/10.1089/ten.tea.2011.0643.

Lee, Ryang Hwa, Byung Chul Kim, Ik Soo Choi, Hanna Kim, Hee Sun Choi, Keun Tak Suh, Yong Chan Bae. & Jin Sup Jung. (2004). "Characterization and Expression Analysis of Mesenchymal Stem Cells from Human Bone Marrow and Adipose Tissue." *Cellular Physiology and Biochemistry*. https://doi.org/10.1159/000080341.

Li, Dong, Peng Zhang, Xiyang Yao, Haiying Li, Haitao Shen, Xiang Li, Jiang Wu. & Xiaocheng Lu. (2018). "Exosomes Derived from MiR-133b-Modified Mesenchymal Stem Cells Promote Recovery after

Spinal Cord Injury." *Frontiers in Neuroscience.* https://doi.org/10.3389/fnins.2018.00845.

Linden, S M van der, Valkenburg, H. A., de Jongh, B. M. & Cats, A. (1984). "The Risk of Developing Ankylosing Spondylitis in HLA-B27 Positive Individuals. A Comparison of Relatives of Spondylitis Patients with the General Population." *Arthritis and Rheumatism.*

Lipsitz, Yonatan Y., William D. Milligan, Ian Fitzpatrick, Evelien Stalmeijer, Suzanne S. Farid, Kah Yong Tan, David Smith., et al. (2017). "A Roadmap for Cost-of-Goods Planning to Guide Economic Production of Cell Therapy Products." *Cytotherapy.* https://doi.org/10.1016/j.jcyt.2017.06.009.

Liu, Gen Zhe, Hirokazu Ishihara, Ryusuke Osada, Tomoatsu Kimura. & Haruo Tsuji. (2001). "Nitric Oxide Mediates the Change of Proteoglycan Synthesis in the Human Lumbar Intervertebral Disc in Response to Hydrostatic Pressure." *Spine.* https://doi.org/10.1097/00007632-200101150-00005.

Louie, P. K., Hassanzadeh, H. & Singh, K. (2014). "Epidemiologic Trends in the Utilization, Demographics, and Cost of Bone Morphogenetic Protein in Spinal Fusions." *Curr Rev Musculoskelet Med*, 7 (3), 177–81. https://doi.org/10.1007/s12178-014-9222-2.

Lu, Kang, Hai yin Li, Kuang Yang, Jun long Wu, Xiao wei Cai, Yue Zhou. & Chang qing Li. (2017). "Exosomes as Potential Alternatives to Stem Cell Therapy for Intervertebral Disc Degeneration: In-Vitro Study on Exosomes in Interaction of Nucleus Pulposus Cells and Bone Marrow Mesenchymal Stem Cells." *Stem Cell Research and Therapy.* https://doi.org/10.1186/s13287-017-0563-9.

Lv, Lin Li, Wei Jun Wu, Ye Feng, Zuo Lin Li, Tao Tao Tang. & Bi Cheng Liu. (2018). "Therapeutic Application of Extracellular Vesicles in Kidney Disease: Promises and Challenges." *Journal of Cellular and Molecular Medicine.* https://doi.org/10.1111/jcmm.13407.

Macfarlane, Gary J., Elaine Thomas, Peter R. Croft, Ann C. Papageorgiou, Malcolm I. V. Jayson. & Alan J. Silman. (1999). "Predictors of Early Improvement in Low Back Pain amongst Consulters to General

Practice: The Influence of Pre-Morbid and Episode-Related Factors." *Pain*. https://doi.org/10.1016/S0304-3959(98)00209-7.

Malik, Nafees N. & Matthew B. Durdy. (2015). "Cell Therapy Landscape: Autologous and Allogeneic Approaches." In *Translational Regenerative Medicine*. https://doi.org/10.1016/B978-0-12-410396-2.00007-4.

Martino, Alberto Di, Alexander R. Vaccaro, Joon Yung Lee, Vincenzo Denaro. & Moe R. Lim. (2005). "Nucleus Pulposus Replacement: Basic Science and Indications for Clinical Use." *Spine*. https://doi.org/10.1097/01.brs.0000174530.88585.32.

Massé, Priscilla G., Maïsha B. Pacifique, Carole C. Tranchant, Barham H. Arjmandi, Karen L. Ericson, Sharon M. Donovan, Edgard Delvin. & Marcel Caissie. (2010). "Bone Metabolic Abnormalities Associated with Well-Controlled Type 1 Diabetes (IDDM) in Young Adult Women: A Disease Complication Often Ignored or Neglected." *Journal of the American College of Nutrition*. https://doi.org/10.1080/07315724.2010.10719859.

Mathivanan, Suresh. & Richard J. Simpson. (2009). "ExoCarta: A Compendium of Exosomal Proteins and RNA." *Proteomics*. https://doi.org/10.1002/pmic.200900351.

Miguel-Beriain, Iñigo de. (2015). "The Ethics of Stem Cells Revisited." *Advanced Drug Delivery Reviews*. https://doi.org/10.1016/j.addr.2014.11.011.

Mo, Irene Fung Ying, Kevin Hak Kong Yip, Wing Keung Chan, Helen Ka Wai Law, Yu Lung Lau. & Godfrey Chi Fung Chan. (2008). "Prolonged Exposure to Bacterial Toxins Downregulated Expression of Toll-like Receptors in Mesenchymal Stromal Cell-Derived Osteoprogenitors." *BMC Cell Biology*. https://doi.org/10.1186/1471-2121-9-52.

Mobbs, Ralph J., Aji Loganathan, Vivian Yeung. & Prashanth J. Rao. (2013). "Indications for Anterior Lumbar Interbody Fusion." *Orthopaedic Surgery*. https://doi.org/10.1111/os.12048.

Mobbs, Ralph J, Kevin Phan, Greg Malham, Kevin Seex. & Prashanth J Rao. (2015). "Lumbar Interbody Fusion: Techniques, Indications and Comparison of Interbody Fusion Options Including PLIF, TLIF, MI-

TLIF, OLIF/ATP, LLIF and ALIF." *Journal of Spine Surgery (Hong Kong)*. https://doi.org/10.3978/j.issn.2414-469X.2015.10.05.

Mohammed, S. & Yu, J. (2018). "Platelet-Rich Plasma Injections: An Emerging Therapy for Chronic Discogenic Low Back Pain." *J Spine Surg*, *4* (1), 115–22. https://doi.org/10.21037/jss.2018.03.04.

Monfett, M., Harrison, J., Boachie-Adjei, K. & Lutz, G. (2016). "Intradiscal Platelet-Rich Plasma (PRP) Injections for Discogenic Low Back Pain: An Update." *Int Orthop*, *40* (6), 1321–28. https://doi.org/10.1007/s00264-016-3178-3.

Morishita, Toru, Kanya Honoki, Hajime Ohgushi, Noriko Kotobuki, Asako Matsushima. & Yoshinori Takakura. (2006). "Tissue Engineering Approach to the Treatment of Bone Tumors: Three Cases of Cultured Bone Grafts Derived from Patients' Mesenchymal Stem Cells." In *Artificial Organs*. https://doi.org/10.1111/j.1525-1594.2006.00190.x.

Murray, Christopher J. L., Jerry Abraham, Mohammed K. Ali, Miriam Alvarado, Charles Atkinson, Larry M. Baddour, David H. Bartels, et al. (2013). "The State of US Health, 1990-2010: Burden of Diseases, Injuries, and Risk Factors." *JAMA - Journal of the American Medical Association*. https://doi.org/10.1001/jama.2013.13805.

Mushahary, Dolly, Andreas Spittler, Cornelia Kasper, Viktoria Weber. & Verena Charwat. (2018). "Isolation, Cultivation, and Characterization of Human Mesenchymal Stem Cells." *Cytometry Part A*. https://doi.org/10.1002/cyto.a.23242.

Naguibneva, Irina, Maya Ameyar-Zazoua, Anna Polesskaya, Slimane Ait-Si-Ali, Reguina Groisman, Mouloud Souidi, Sylvain Cuvellier. & Annick Harel-Bellan. (2006). "The MicroRNA MiR-181 Targets the Homeobox Protein Hox-A11 during Mammalian Myoblast Differentiation." *Nature Cell Biology*. https://doi.org/10.1038/ncb1373.

Navani, A., Manchikanti, L., Albers, S. L., Latchaw, R. E., Sanapati, J., Kaye, A. D., Atluri, S., et al. (2019). "Responsible, Safe, and Effective Use of Biologics in the Management of Low Back Pain: American Society of Interventional Pain Physicians (ASIPP) Guidelines." *Pain Physician* 22 (1S): S1–74. https://www.ncbi.nlm.nih.gov/pubmed/30717500.

Neviani, Paolo. & Muller Fabbri. (2015). "Exosomic MicroRNAs in the Tumor Microenvironment." *Frontiers in Medicine*. https://doi.org/10.3389/fmed.2015.00047.

Noh, K. C., Liu, X. N., Zhuan, Z., Yang, C. J., Kim, Y. T., Lee, G. W., Choi, K. H. & Kim, K. O. (2018). "Leukocyte-Poor Platelet-Rich Plasma-Derived Growth Factors Enhance Human Fibroblast Proliferation *In Vitro*." *Clin Orthop Surg*, *10* (2), 240–47. https://doi.org/10.4055/cios.2018.10.2.240.

Noriega, David C., Francisco Ardura, Rubén Hernández-Ramajo, Miguel Ángel Martín-Ferrero, Israel Sánchez-Lite, Borja Toribio, Mercedes Alberca., et al. (2017). "Intervertebral Disc Repair by Allogeneic Mesenchymal Bone Marrow Cells: A Randomized Controlled Trial." *Transplantation*. https://doi.org/10.1097/TP.0000000000001484.

Oh, Min. & Jacques E. Nör. (2015). "The Perivascular Niche and Self-Renewal of Stem Cells." *Frontiers in Physiology*. https://doi.org/10.3389/fphys.2015.00367.

Orozco, Lluis, Robert Soler, Carles Morera, Mercedes Alberca, Ana Sánchez. & Javier García-Sancho. (2011). "Intervertebral Disc Repair by Autologous Mesenchymal Bone Marrow Cells: A Pilot Study." *Transplantation*. https://doi.org/10.1097/TP.0b013e3182298a15.

Oryan, Ahmad, Amir Kamali, Ali Moshirib. & Mohamadreza Baghaban Eslaminejad. (2017). "Role of Mesenchymal Stem Cells in Bone Regenerative Medicine: What Is the Evidence?" *Cells Tissues Organs*. https://doi.org/10.1159/000469704.

Pap, E., Pállinger, É, Pásztói, M. & Falus, A. (2009). "Highlights of a New Type of Intercellular Communication: Microvesicle-Based Information Transfer." *Inflammation Research*. https://doi.org/10.1007/s00011-008-8210-7.

Park, Sung Bae. & Chun Kee Chung. (2011). "Strategies of Spinal Fusion on Osteoporotic Spine." *Journal of Korean Neurosurgical Society*. https://doi.org/10.3340/jkns.2011.49.6.317.

Pirvu, T. N., Schroeder, J. E., Peroglio, M., Verrier, S., Kaplan, L., Richards, R. G., Alini, M. & Grad, S. (2014). "Platelet-Rich Plasma Induces

Annulus Fibrosus Cell Proliferation and Matrix Production." *Eur Spine J*, *23* (4), 745–53. https://doi.org/10.1007/s00586-014-3198-x.

Pisitkun, Trairak, Rong Fong Shen. & Mark A. Knepper. (2004). "Identification and Proteomic Profiling of Exosomes in Human Urine." *Proceedings of the National Academy of Sciences of the United States of America*. https://doi.org/10.1073/pnas.0403453101.

Priyadarshani, P., Li, Y. & Yao, L. (2016). "Advances in Biological Therapy for Nucleus Pulposus Regeneration." *Osteoarthritis and Cartilage*. https://doi.org/10.1016/j.joca.2015.08.014.

Pull Ter Gunne, Albert F., Allard J. F. Hosman, David B. Cohen, Michael Schuetz, Drmed Habil, Cees J. H. M. Van Laarhoven. & Joost J. Van Middendorp. (2012). "A Methodological Systematic Review on Surgical Site Infections Following Spinal Surgery: Part 1: Risk Factors." *Spine*. https://doi.org/10.1097/BRS.0b013e31825bfca8.

Raicevic, Gordana, Redouane Rouas, Mehdi Najar, Patrick Stordeur, Hicham Id Boufker, Dominique Bron, Philippe Martiat, Michel Goldman, Michel T. Nevessignsky. & Laurence Lagneaux. (2010). "Inflammation Modifies the Pattern and the Function of Toll-like Receptors Expressed by Human Mesenchymal Stromal Cells." *Human Immunology*. https://doi.org/10.1016/j.humimm.2009.12.005.

Ratajczak, M. Z., Kucia, M., Jadczyk, T., Greco, N. J., Wojakowski, W., Tendera, M. & Ratajczak, J. (2012). "Pivotal Role of Paracrine Effects in Stem Cell Therapies in Regenerative Medicine: Can We Translate Stem Cell-Secreted Paracrine Factors and Microvesicles into Better Therapeutic Strategies." *Leukemia*. https://doi.org/10.1038/leu.2011.389.

Richardson, Stephen M., Rachael V. Walker, Siân Parker, Nicholas P. Rhodes, John A. Hunt, Anthony J. Freemont. & Judith A. Hoyland. (2006). "Intervertebral Disc Cell-Mediated Mesenchymal Stem Cell Differentiation." *Stem Cells*. https://doi.org/10.1634/stemcells.2005-0205.

Risbud, Makarand V. & Irving M. Shapiro. (2014). "Role of Cytokines in Intervertebral Disc Degeneration: Pain and Disc Content." *Nature Reviews Rheumatology*. https://doi.org/10.1038/nrrheum.2013.160.

Sakaguchi, Yusuke, Ichiro Sekiya, Kazuyoshi Yagishita. & Takeshi Muneta. (2005). "Comparison of Human Stem Cells Derived from Various Mesenchymal Tissues: Superiority of Synovium as a Cell Source." *Arthritis and Rheumatism*. https://doi.org/10.1002/art.21212.

Sakai, Daisuke, Joji Mochida, Toru Iwashina, Akihiko Hiyama, Hiroko Omi, Masaaki Imai, Tomoko Nakai, Kiyoshi Ando. & Tomomitsu Hotta. (2006). "Regenerative Effects of Transplanting Mesenchymal Stem Cells Embedded in Atelocollagen to the Degenerated Intervertebral Disc." *Biomaterials*. https://doi.org/10.1016/j.biomaterials.2005.06.038.

Sakai, Daisuke, Joji Mochida, Yukihiro Yamamoto, Takeshi Nomura, Masahiko Okuma, Kazuhiro Nishimura, Tomoko Nakai, Kiyoshi Ando. & Tomomitsu Hotta. (2003). "Transplantation of Mesenchymal Stem Cells Embedded in Atelocollagen® Gel to the Intervertebral Disc: A Potential Therapeutic Model for Disc Degeneration." *Biomaterials*. https://doi.org/10.1016/S0142-9612(03)00222-9.

Salamanna, F., Veronesi, F., Maglio, M., Della Bella, E., Sartori, M. & Fini, M. (2015). "New and Emerging Strategies in Platelet-Rich Plasma Application in Musculoskeletal Regenerative Procedures: General Overview on Still Open Questions and Outlook." *Biomed Res Int*, 846045. https://doi.org/10.1155/2015/846045.

Satake, Kotaro, Tokumi Kanemura, Akiyuki Matsumoto, Hidetoshi Yamaguchi. & Yoshimoto Ishikawa. (2013). "Predisposing Factors for Surgical Site Infection of Spinal Instrumentation Surgery for Diabetes Patients." *European Spine Journal*. https://doi.org/10.1007/s00586-013-2783-8.

Siekevitz, P. (1972). "Biological Membranes: The Dynamics of Their Organization." *Annual Review of Physiology*. https://doi.org/10.1146/annurev.ph.34.030172.001001.

Simaria, Ana S., Sally Hassan, Hemanthram Varadaraju, Jon Rowley, Kim Warren, Philip Vanek. & Suzanne S. Farid. (2014). "Allogeneic Cell Therapy Bioprocess Economics and Optimization: Single-Use Cell Expansion Technologies." *Biotechnology and Bioengineering*. https://doi.org/10.1002/bit.25008.

Simental-Mendia, M., Vilchez-Cavazos, F., Garcia-Garza, R., Lara-Arias, J., Montes-de-Oca-Luna, R., Said-Fernandez, S. & Martinez-Rodriguez, H. G. (2018). "The Matrix Synthesis and Anti-Inflammatory Effect of Autologous Leukocyte-Poor Platelet Rich Plasma in Human Cartilage Explants." *Histol Histopathol*, *33* (6), 609–18. https://doi.org/10.14670/HH-11-961.

Simons, Mikael. & Graça Raposo. (2009). "Exosomes - Vesicular Carriers for Intercellular Communication." *Current Opinion in Cell Biology*. https://doi.org/10.1016/j.ceb.2009.03.007.

Smith, R. Lane, Dennis R. Carter. & David J. Schurman. (2004). "Pressure and Shear Differentially Alter Human Articular Chondrocyte Metabolism: A Review." In *Clinical Orthopaedics and Related Research*.

Taghavi, Cyrus E., Kwang Bok Lee, Gun Keorochana, Shiau Tzu Tzeng, Jeong Hyun Yoo. & Jeffrey C. Wang. (2010). "Bone Morphogenetic Protein-2 and Bone Marrow Aspirate with Allograft as Alternatives to Autograft in Instrumented Revision Posterolateral Lumbar Spinal Fusion: A Minimum Two-Year Follow-up Study." *Spine*. https://doi.org/10.1097/BRS.0b013e3181bb5203.

Takahashi, Shinji, Akinobu Suzuki, Hiromitsu Toyoda, Hidetomi Terai, Sho Dohzono, Kentarou Yamada, Tomiya Matsumoto., et al. (2013). "Characteristics of Diabetes Associated with Poor Improvements in Clinical Outcomes after Lumbar Spine Surgery." *Spine*. https://doi.org/10.1097/BRS.0b013e318273583a.

Tanaka, Youhei, Hidenobu Kamohara, Kouichi Kinoshita, Junji Kurashige, Takatsugu Ishimoto, Masaaki Iwatsuki, Masayuki Watanabe. & Hideo Baba. (2013). "Clinical Impact of Serum Exosomal MicroRNA-21 as a Clinical Biomarker in Human Esophageal Squamous Cell Carcinoma." *Cancer*. https://doi.org/10.1002/cncr.27895.

Tetta, Ciro, Stefania Bruno, Valentina Fonsato, Maria Chiara Deregibus. & Giovanni Camussi. (2011). "The Role of Microvesicles in Tissue Repair." *Organogenesis*. https://doi.org/10.4161/org.7.2.15782.

Théry, Clotilde, Matias Ostrowski. & Elodie Segura. (2009). "Membrane Vesicles as Conveyors of Immune Responses." *Nature Reviews Immunology*. https://doi.org/10.1038/nri2567.

Tian, Ye, Wen Yuan, Nobuyuki Fujita, Jianru Wang, Hua Wang, Irving M. Shapiro. & Makarand V. Risbud. (2013). "Inflammatory Cytokines Associated with Degenerative Disc Disease Control Aggrecanase-1 (ADAMTS-4) Expression in Nucleus Pulposus Cells through MAPK and NF-KB." *American Journal of Pathology*. https://doi.org/10.1016/j.ajpath.2013.02.037.

Tulder, Maurits W. van, Bart W. Koes. & Lex M. Bouter. (1997). "Conservative Treatment of Acute and Chronic Nonspecific Low Back Pain." *Spine*. https://doi.org/10.1097/00007632-199709150-00012.

Urban, Jill P. G., Stanton Smith. & Jeremy C. T. Fairbank. (2004). "Nutrition of the Intervertebral Disc." *Spine*. https://doi.org/10.1097/01.brs.0000146499.97948.52.

Vadalà, Gianluca, Fabrizio Russo, Luca Ambrosio, Mattia Loppini. & Vincenzo Denaro. (2016). "Stem Cells Sources for Intervertebral Disc Regeneration." *World Journal of Stem Cells*. https://doi.org/10.4252/wjsc.v8.i5.185.

Valenti, Roberta, Veronica Huber, Manuela Iero, Paola Filipazzi, Giorgio Parmiani. & Licia Rivoltini. (2007). "Tumor-Released Microvesicles as Vehicles of Immunosuppression." *Cancer Research*. https://doi.org/10.1158/0008-5472.CAN-07-0520.

Vergroesen, P. P. A., Kingma, I., Emanuel, K. S., Hoogendoorn, R. J. W., Welting, T. J., van Royen, B. J., van Dieën, J. H. & Smit, T. H. (2015). "Mechanics and Biology in Intervertebral Disc Degeneration: A Vicious Circle." *Osteoarthritis and Cartilage*. https://doi.org/10.1016/j.joca.2015.03.028.

Vizoso, Francisco J., Noemi Eiro, Sandra Cid, Jose Schneider. & Roman Perez-Fernandez. (2017). "Mesenchymal Stem Cell Secretome: Toward Cell-Free Therapeutic Strategies in Regenerative Medicine." *International Journal of Molecular Sciences*. https://doi.org/10.3390/ijms18091852.

Vlassov, Alexander V., Susan Magdaleno, Robert Setterquist. & Rick Conrad. (2012). "Exosomes: Current Knowledge of Their Composition, Biological Functions, and Diagnostic and Therapeutic Potentials." *Biochimica et Biophysica Acta - General Subjects.* https://doi.org/10.1016/ j.bbagen.2012.03.017.

Waddell, G. (1987). "A New Clinical Model for the Treatment of Low-Back Pain." *Spine.* https://doi.org/10.1097/00007632-198709000-00002.

Wang, Hai, Yue Zhou, Bo Huang, Lan Tao Liu, Ming Han Liu, Jian Wang, Chang Qing Li, Zhen Feng Zhang, Tong Wei Chu. & Cheng Jie Xiong. (2014). "Utilization of Stem Cells in Alginate for Nucleus Pulposus Tissue Engineering." *Tissue Engineering - Part A.* https://doi.org/ 10.1089/ten.tea.2012.0703.

Wang, Peng, Yuxi Li, Lin Huang, Jiewen Yang, Rui Yang, Wen Deng, Biling Liang., et al. (2014). "Effects and Safety of Allogenic Mesenchymal Stem Cell Intravenous Infusion in Active Ankylosing Spondylitis Patients Who Failed NSAIDs: A 20-Week Clinical Trial." *Cell Transplantation.* https://doi.org/10.3727/096368913X667727.

Wang, S. Z., Fan, W. M., Jia, J., Ma, L. Y., Yu, J. B. & Wang, C. (2018). "Is Exclusion of Leukocytes from Platelet-Rich Plasma (PRP) a Better Choice for Early Intervertebral Disc Regeneration?" *Stem Cell Res Ther*, 9 (1), 199. https://doi.org/10.1186/s13287-018-0937-7.

Ward, Michael M., Atul Deodhar, Lianne S. Gensler, Maureen Dubreuil, David Yu, Muhammad Asim Khan, Nigil Haroon., et al. (2019). "2019 Update of the American College of Rheumatology/Spondylitis Association of America/Spondyloarthritis Research and Treatment Network Recommendations for the Treatment of Ankylosing Spondylitis and Nonradiographic Axial Spondyloarthritis." *Arthritis and Rheumatology.* https://doi.org/10.1002/art.41042.

Wasterlain, A. S., Braun, H. J., Harris, A. H., Kim, H. J. & Dragoo, J. L. (2013). "The Systemic Effects of Platelet-Rich Plasma Injection." *Am J Sports Med*, 41 (1), 186–93. https://doi.org/10.1177/ 0363546512466383.

Waterman, Ruth S., Suzanne L. Tomchuck, Sarah L. Henkle. & Aline M. Betancourt. (2010). "A New Mesenchymal Stem Cell (MSC) Paradigm:

Polarization into a pro-Inflammatory MSC1 or an Immunosuppressive MSC2 Phenotype." *PLoS ONE.* https://doi.org/10.1371/journal.pone.0010088.

Weiss, K R. (2015). "'To B(MP-2) or Not To B(MP-2)' or 'Much Ado About Nothing': Are Orthobiologics in Tumor Surgery Worth the Risks?" *Clin Cancer Res, 21* (13), 2889–91. https://doi.org/10.1158/1078-0432.CCR-14-3069.

Willis, Gareth R., Stella Kourembanas. & Alex Mitsialis, S. (2017). "Toward Exosome-Based Therapeutics: Isolation, Heterogeneity, and Fit-for-Purpose Potency." *Frontiers in Cardiovascular Medicine.* https://doi.org/10.3389/fcvm.2017.00063.

Wong, Rebecca S. Y. (2015). "Role of Stem Cells in Spondyloarthritis: Pathogenesis, Treatment and Complications." *Human Immunology.* https://doi.org/10.1016/j.humimm.2015.09.038.

Wu, J., Zhou, J., Liu, C., Zhang, J., Xiong, W., Lv, Y., Liu, R., et al. (2017). "A Prospective Study Comparing Platelet-Rich Plasma and Local Anesthetic (LA)/Corticosteroid in Intra-Articular Injection for the Treatment of Lumbar Facet Joint Syndrome." *Pain Pract, 17* (7), 914–24. https://doi.org/10.1111/papr.12544.

Wu, Sharon F., Nicole Noren Hooten, David W. Freeman, Nicolle A. Mode, Alan B. Zonderman. & Michele K. Evans. (2020). "Extracellular Vesicles in Diabetes Mellitus Induce Alterations in Endothelial Cell Morphology and Migration." *Journal of Translational Medicine.* https://doi.org/10.1186/s12967-020-02398-6.

Wubbolts, Richard, Rachel S. Leckie, Peter T. M. Veenhuizen, Guenter Schwarzmann, Wiebke Möbius, Joerg Hoernschemeyer, Jan Willem Slot, Hans J. Geuze. & Willem Stoorvogel. (2003). "Proteomic and Biochemical Analyses of Human B Cell-Derived Exosomes: Potential Implications for Their Function and Multivesicular Body Formation." *Journal of Biological Chemistry.* https://doi.org/10.1074/jbc.M207550200.

Wukich, Dane K. (2015). "Diabetes and Its Negative Impact on Outcomes in Orthopaedic Surgery." *World Journal of Orthopaedics.* https://doi.org/10.5312/wjo.v6.i3.331.

Xia, Chen, Zhongyou Zeng, Bin Fang, Min Tao, Chenhui Gu, Lin Zheng, Wang, Y., et al. (2019). "Mesenchymal Stem Cell-Derived Exosomes Ameliorate Intervertebral Disc Degeneration via Anti-Oxidant and Anti-Inflammatory Effects." *Free Radical Biology and Medicine*. https://doi.org/10.1016/j.freeradbiomed.2019.07.026.

Yaari, L., Dolev, A. & Haviv, B. (2019). "[Platelet Rich Plasma Injection as Treatment for Rotator Cuff Tendinopathy and as an Augmentation for Rotator Cuff Repair]." *Harefuah*, *158* (6), 395–97. https://www.ncbi.nlm.nih.gov/pubmed/31215193.

Yamakawa, J., Hashimoto, J., Takano, M. & Takagi, M. (2017). "The Bone Regeneration Using Bone Marrow Stromal Cells with Moderate Concentration Platelet-Rich Plasma in Femoral Segmental Defect of Rats." *Open Orthop J*, *11*, 1–11. https://doi.org/10.2174/1874325001711010001.

Yamashita, Takuma, Yuki Takahashi, Makiya Nishikawa. & Yoshinobu Takakura. (2016). "Effect of Exosome Isolation Methods on Physicochemical Properties of Exosomes and Clearance of Exosomes from the Blood Circulation." *European Journal of Pharmaceutics and Biopharmaceutics*. https://doi.org/10.1016/j.ejpb.2015.10.017.

Yamashita, Takuma, Yuki Takahashi. & Yoshinobu Takakura. (2018). "Possibility of Exosome-Based Therapeutics and Challenges in Production of Exosomes Eligible for Therapeutic Application." *Biological and Pharmaceutical Bulletin*. https://doi.org/10.1248/bpb.b18-00133.

Yeh Yeo, Ronne Wee, Ruenn Chai, Kok Hian. & Sai Kiang. (2013). "Exosome: A Novel and Safer Therapeutic Refinement of Mesenchymal Stem Cell." *Exosomes and Microvesicles*. https://doi.org/10.5772/57460.

Yoshikawa, Takafumi, Yurito Ueda, Kiyoshi Miyazaki, Munehisa Koizumi. & Yoshinori Takakura. (2010). "Disc Regeneration Therapy Using Marrow Mesenchymal Cell Transplantation: A Report of Two Case Studies." *Spine*. https://doi.org/10.1097/ BRS.0b013e3181cd2cf4.

Yousef, Mohamed Abdelhamid Ali, Giovanni Andrea La Maida. & Bernardo Misaggi. (2017). "Long-Term Radiological and Clinical

Outcomes after Using Bone Marrow Mesenchymal Stem Cells Concentrate Obtained with Selective Retention Cell Technology in Posterolateral Spinal Fusion." *Spine.* https://doi.org/10.1097/BRS.0000000000002255.

Zhang, Baolong, Linfei Xu, Naiqiang Zhuo. & Jieliang Shen. (2017). "Resveratrol Protects against Mitochondrial Dysfunction through Autophagy Activation in Human Nucleus Pulposus Cells." *Biochemical and Biophysical Research Communications.* https://doi.org/10.1016/j.bbrc.2017.09.015.

Zhang, Jieyuan, Junjie Guan, Xin Niu, Guowen Hu, Shangchun Guo, Qing Li, Zongping Xie, Changqing Zhang. & Yang Wang. (2015). "Exosomes Released from Human Induced Pluripotent Stem Cells-Derived MSCs Facilitate Cutaneous Wound Healing by Promoting Collagen Synthesis and Angiogenesis." *Journal of Translational Medicine.* https://doi.org/10.1186/s12967-015-0417-0.

Zhang, Xin, Yong Ma, Xin Fu, Qiang Liu, Zhenxing Shao, Linghui Dai, Yanbin Pi., et al. (2016). "Runx2-Modified Adipose-Derived Stem Cells Promote Tendon Graft Integration in Anterior Cruciate Ligament Reconstruction." *Scientific Reports.* https://doi.org/10.1038/srep19073.

Zhang, Yin Gang, Xiong Guo, Peng Xu, Long Li Kang. & Jun Li. (2005). "Bone Mesenchymal Stem Cells Transplanted into Rabbit Intervertebral Discs Can Increase Proteoglycans." *Clinical Orthopaedics and Related Research.* https://doi.org/10.1097/ 01.blo.0000146534.31120.cf.

Zhuang, Guanglei, Xiumin Wu, Zhaoshi Jiang, Ian Kasman, Jenny Yao, Yinghui Guan, Jason Oeh, et al. (2012). "Tumour-Secreted MiR-9 Promotes Endothelial Cell Migration and Angiogenesis by Activating the JAK-STAT Pathway." *EMBO Journal.* https://doi.org/10.1038/emboj.2012.183.

In: The Fundamentals of Spine Surgery
Editor: Tim Bachmeier

ISBN: 978-1-53618-570-6
© 2020 Nova Science Publishers, Inc.

Chapter 2

FUSION RATE AFTER LLIF PROCEDURES IN LUMBAR ADULT DEFORMITIES: THE STATE OF ART

Andrea Perna[1,2], MD, Alessandro Ramieri[3],*, MD, PhD, Luca Ricciardi[4,5], MD, Luca Proietti[1,2], MD, Massimo Miscusi[5], PhD, Georgios Bakaloudis[6], MD, Domenico Alessandro Santagada[1,2], MD, Francesco Ciro Tamburrelli[1,2], MD, Antonino Raco[5], PhD and Giuseppe Costanzo[3]

[1]Rome, Italy, IRCCS Foundation Agostino Gemelli
[2]Rome, Italy, Orthopaedics and Traumatology, Catholic University
[3]Rome, Italy, Faculty of Pharmacy and Medicine,
Dpt Orthopaedics and Traumatology, University "La Sapienza"
[4]Tricase (Lecce), Italy Cardinal G. Panico, Neurosurgery
[5]Rome, Italy, Dpt NESMOS Sant'Andrea Hospital University
"La Sapienza"
[6]Rome Italy, Spinal Surgery, Guarnieri Hospital

---

* Corresponding Author's E-mail: alexramieri@libero.it.

Abstract

Purpose: In few studies, fusion rate in XLIF, assessed by CT scan, ranged between 85 and 93%. Aims of our study were: - estimate fusion by 3D CT scan in XLIFs applied only in adult lumbar deformities; - evaluate clinical results related to fusion.

Materials and Methods: 193 XLIFs (147 titanium, 51peeks) performed in 79 adult degenerative lumbar scoliosis and 44 spondylolisthesis were evaluated by 3D CT scan at least 1 yr follow-up, distinguishing complete fusion (F), probably fusion (PF) and pseudoarthrosis (P), as well as subsidence and/or mobilization. Clinical results on VAS and ODI were compared in relation to the degree of fusion. Different bone grafts were used: bovine bone mineral and collagen; calcium phosphate granules or paste; paste of demineralized bone matrix.

Results: We recorded 75% of F, 19% of PF and 6% P. Pseudoarthrosis involved 7 titanium and 6 PEEK cages. Particularly exposed to subsidence or settling were middle cages in 3-level XLIFs. The worst clinical condition concerned pseudoarthrosis with loss of correction.

Conclusions: The fusion rate in our case series, consisting of only adult deformities, at one year follow-up, was lower than those reported in the literature. Pseudoarthrosis, cage settling and loss of lumbar lordosis correction were factors that negatively affected our clinical outcomes.

Keywords: spine, fusion rate, LLIF, XLIF, adult spinal deformity, minimally, invasive spine surgery

1. Introduction

Nowadays, lumbar spine degenerative disease (LSDD) associated with adult spinal deformity (ASD) represents a widespread condition, increasingly requiring surgical treatment [1]. Despite the advance of technologies and biomaterial sciences applied to instrumentation and mini-invasive surgical (MIS) techniques, interbody fusion procedures along with open or percutaneous posterior trans-pedicle screws fixation (PTSF) still represent the gold standard treatment of different lumbar degenerative disorders [2].

The aim of using interbody devices would be to restore and maintain a normal disc space and segmental lordosis, to increase the mechanical stability and to restore the native anatomy of the spinal segment, eventually influencing the global spine alignment. The stretching of the anterior column, by distracting the segment using either direct or indirect techniques, is also known as "ligamentotaxis". When associated to PTSF it allows to reach a stable mechanical construct, theoretically resulting in segmental immobilization and higher chances for fusion [2-3]. To obtain interbody fusion a proper vertebral end-plate preparation, removing discal fragments and exposing the cortical rim, is a mandatory step for fostering the ossification throughout the discal space, thus semgnetal somatodesis. [4]. Primary mechanical stability of the treated segment, provided by the instrumentation, is supposed to facilitate the fusion process [2, 4]. However, multiple factors can influence the interbody fusion process, including patient related factors, cage material/design, bone graft material, and surgical technique [4].

The goals of surgical treatment in ASD should include spinal cord decompression, sagittal and coronal balance restoration and a solid secondary fusion (no longer dependent from the instrumentation system), then improving patients health-related quality of life [1]. Different surgical techniques have been proposed during the last decades, demonstrated as able to result in a solid interbody fusion. However, the concept that the least invasive technique should be always performed has to be preferred has been progressively accepted and validated in the scientific Literature [2]. The advantages of MIS procedure applied to the spinal disorders, compared with the open procedures, have been widely reported. Among these, we need to highlight the reduced intraoperative blood loss and perioperative pain rate, the minimal injury of soft tissues, the possibility for an earlier mobilization, and shorter hospitalization [5].

Among MIS procedures, Lateral Lumbar Interbody Fusion (LLIF) represents a safe, well tolerated and reliable alternative technique to posterolateral procedures, which are still preferred by most of spinal surgeons to perform lumbar interbody fusion [2] LLIF consists in a retroperitoneal direct spinal lateral access that allows to insert a large footprint cage, to perform an and wider accurate discectomy and end-plates preparation, bilateral annular ligament release, indirect decompression of neural foraminal and nerve roots, and coronal/sagittal deformity correction, preservating the posterior elements, such as ligaments and zygoapofisal joints [6]. Furthermore, it provides a strong primary stability, which leads to a solid interbody fusion. Althogh in properly selected cases, percutaneous PTSF alone could ensure an imobilization grade eventually leading to fusion [7], LLIF allows to insert a higher amount of bone graft, compared with conventional posterior lumbar interbody fusion devices, further facilitating the ossification process (Figure 1) [8-9].

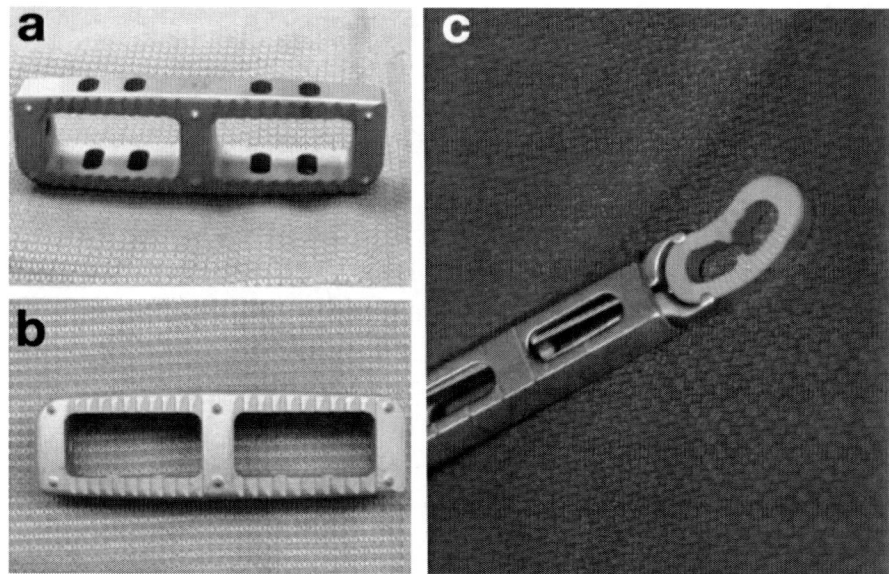

Figure 1. a,b, Titanium cage used in XLIF procedure. It is possible observe the difference of cage footprint and the space reserved to bone graft compared with 1:1 TLIF cage shown in figure c.

Although the fusion rate is frequently reported as an outcome in clinical studies on lumbar fusion, a general consensus on its evaluation after a LLIF is still missing [10-11]. Although different methods were reported in radiographic studies, but the presence of cancellous bone bridges between two adjacent vertebral endplates, with no longer evidence of cortical rim, has been proposed as a pathognomonic sign of interbody fusion [12-13]. Computer tomography (CT), with fine-cuts and multiplanar 3D images reconstruction, still represents the gold standard for the evaluation of interbody fusion [11].

There are few studies reporting CT scan-assessed fusion rate after LLIF assessed. We aimed to investigate the fusion rate using 3D CT scan, in patients with ASD who underwent LLIF and percutaneous PTSF, measuring any existing clinical radiological correlation.

2. METHODS

2.1. Study Design and Settings

The present investigation consists in a retrospective multicentre analysis collecting radiographical data from the institutional Picture archiving and communication system (PACS), clinical and functional data from outpatient medical records, in a time range from January 2016 to December 2018. Clinical data were retrieved at the following observation times: preoperatively, 1 month, 6 months, and 1 year after surgery.The present study matched national ethical standards and the Helsinki Convention. Data collection was approved by the IRB of the authors' affiliated institutions. Written informed consent for scientific purposes and clinical data collection was obtained according to institutional protocols.

2.2. Inclusion and Exclusion Criteria

All patients affected by ASD who underwent LLIF (on one or more levels) and percutaneous PTSF were considered as eligible for the present study. Only patient with complete radiographical and clinical data set and at least 12 months of follow up were included. Exclusion criteria were: (I) age > 70; (II) severe osteoporosis (t-score < 2.0); (III) previous instrumented spine surgery; (IV) presence of rheumatic disease (e.g., Ankylosing spondylitis, rheumatoid arthritis, diffuse idiopathic skeletal hyperostosis, DISH); (V) postoperative spine infection; (VI) metastatic and/or primary neoplastic vertebral lesions; (VII) post-traumatic deformity; (VIII) Stand-alone procedure without additional posterior instrumentation.

2.3. Surgical Technique

The LLIF procedure, performed according Ozgur et al. [14] using an intraoperative neuromonitoring system M5 (Nuvasive, San Diego, CA, US) and conventional C-arm fluoroscopy (BV Pulsera, Koninklijke Philips N.V.), represented the first surgical step in all included patients. All procedures were performed under general anaesthesia, in lateral decubitus with a slight flexion of the hip by two surgical teams. Instrumentation system XLIF (Nuvasive, San Diego, CA, US) was used in all cases. A retroperitoneal lateral approach was done using a dedicated tubular retractor for psoas splitting. After identification of the disc space a complete and accurate discectomy was performed under fluoroscopic guidance. Particular attention was reserved to release the contralateral annulus, and preparation of the vertebral end-plates avoiding their violations. An appropriate sized cage was inserted under AP fluoroscopic guidance. All cages implanted were made by PolyEther Ether Ketone (PEEK) or titanium and were filled with grafts materials. Three type of bone graft were used: Attrax™ (Nuvasive, San Diego, CA, US), ß tricalcium-phosphate and demineralized bone matrix.

In the second surgical step a percutaneous posterior fixation in prone position was performed using bilateral titanium pedicle screws and rods (Precept, Nuvasive, San Diego, CA, US) in all enrolled patients. No patients underwent any direct open or mini-invasive laminectomy decompression.

2.4. Clinical Outcomes

Functional evaluation in all follow-up visits was assessed by Oswestry Disability Index (ODI) score. Clinical evaluation was performed by a ten itemized Visual analogue scale (VAS) for back pain. Perioperative complications were also recorded.

2.5. Radiological Outcomes

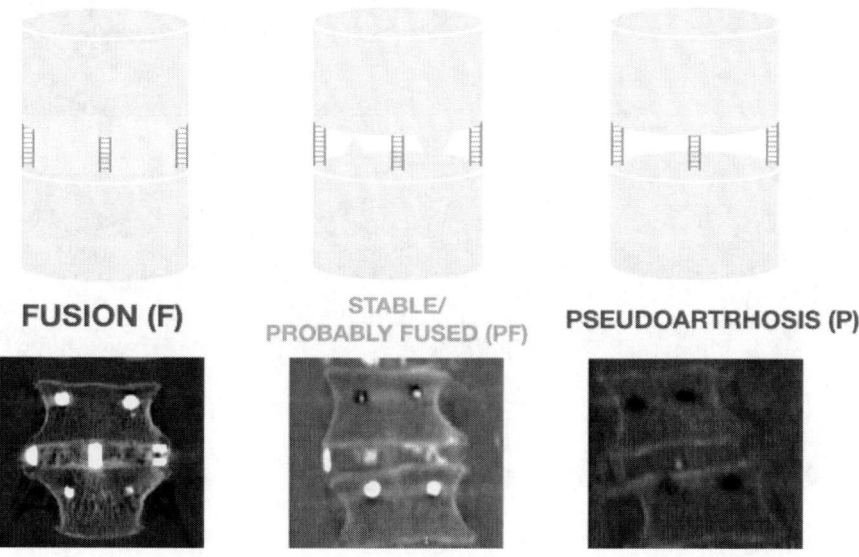

Figure 2. The figure showed the Berjano et al. [15] classification as mentioned in the text. On the top of the image was possible to observe the schematic representation of Berjano's classification, while on the bottom of the figure were reported coronal CT scan images of a fused, probably fused and pseudarthrosis vertebral segment.

All patients enrolled in the present investigation underwent a standard radiologic follow up consisting in: immediately post-operative, 3 and 6 months lumbar spine plain X-Ray in latero-lateral and anteroposterior views; a lumbar spine CT scans with triplanar and 3D images reconstruction 12 months after surgery. Radiologic images were retrieved and independently reviewed by three authors, using PACS and a dedicated workstation. The fusion rate was evaluated according Berjano et al. classification [15] based on CT scan images (Figure 2).

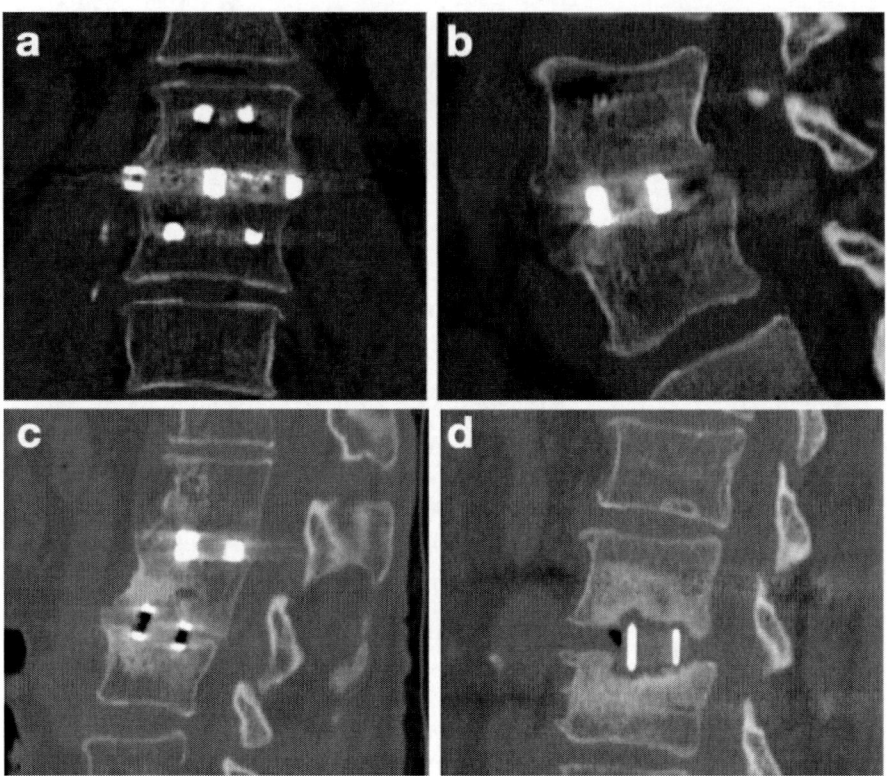

Figure 3. a,b, Coronal and sagittal CT scan images of a complete fused segment. It was possible to observe the presence of BB intra- and extra cage in both figure. c, Sagittal CT scan image of a fused segment with cage subsidence and loss of lumbar lordosis. d, Sagittal CT scan images of a patient belonging to the pseudarthrosis group; a cage subsidence could be observed.

Patients with presence of BB in the interbody space connecting two contiguous vertebral endplate were considered fused (F) (Figure 3 a,b). When interbody space BB were incomplete and a minimal radiolucency was observed at only one graft-endplate interface without instrumentation loosening the patients were considered stable, probably fused (PF). When a complete radiolucency in both interfaces with graft resorption were detected or an instrumentation (cage and screws) loosening was observed, pseudoarthrosis (P) occurred. Based on CT scan images the cage subsidence rate was recorded. Cage subsidence (CS) was defined as the presence of a sinking of the cage in the superior or inferior vertebral endplate > of 3 mm (Figure 3, c,d). In all patients included, spinopelvic parameters (Pelvic index, PI; Pelvic Tilt, PT, Sacral Slope, SS; Lumbar Lordosis, LL) were recorded on whole spine plain radiographs in antero-posterior (AP) and lateral views preoperatively, immediately postoperatively and 12 months after surgery.

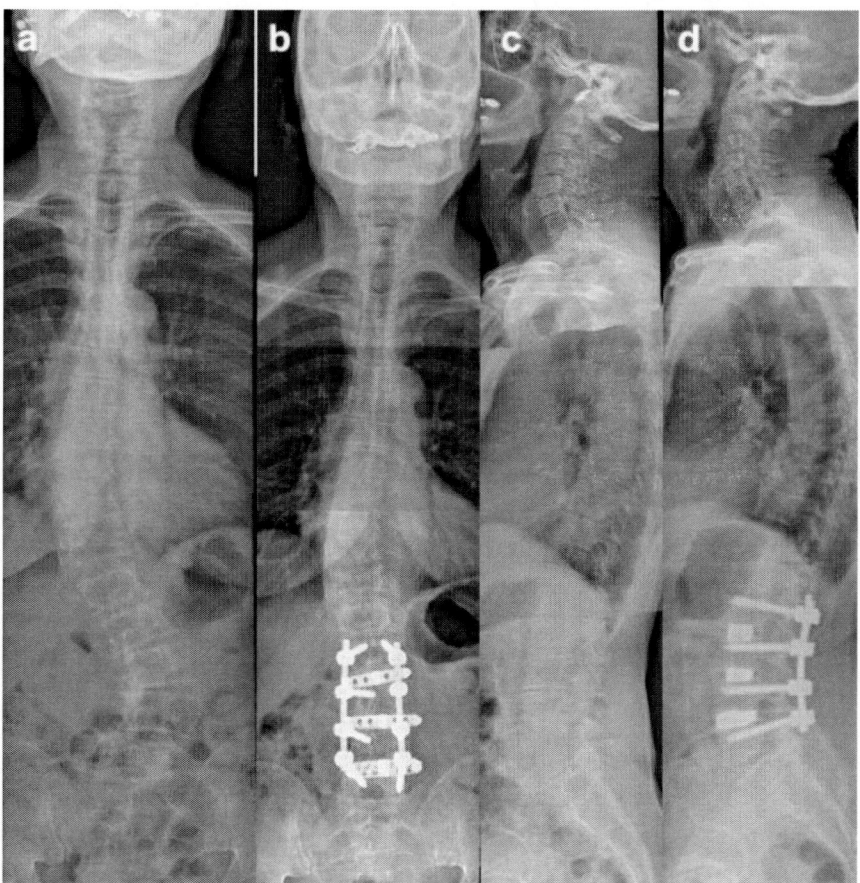

Figure 4. a,c, Preoperative full spine standing X-Ray in a patient with adult degenerative lumbar scoliosis. b,d, Postoperative X-Ray showing the deformity correction on coronal plane and a good sagittal balance after cage placement at level L2-L3,L3-L4 and L4-L5 and PTSF L2-L5.

The mean disc angle variation according methods decribed by Barone et al. [1] was also recorded preoperatively, immediately postoperatively and 12 months after surgery on plain radiographs (Figure 4).

2.6. Statistical Analysis

Statistical analysis were performed using a dedicated software (SPSS v.19.0, SPSS Inc.; Chicago, IL). The Mann–Whitney U-test was used for two independent ordinal variables. The Wilcoxon signed-rank test was used for two dependent ordinal variables. The significance was established for a value of $p < 0.05$. The inter-rater reliability (IRR) between the three evaluators was calculated using a Fleiss' kappa statistic. Data are reported as means and standard deviations (SD) and only one decimal digit was reported, as rounded up. Data normality was tested before performing other statistical analysis.

3. RESULTS

3.1. Participants

Out of the 192 patients considered for eligibility, 123 were finally included in the present investigation, according to the aforementioned inclusion criteria. The mean age was 61.4 (± 8.3) years, the male/female ratio was 1:1.7 (M: 46; F: 77), and the mean follow-up time was 18.8 (± 1.1) years.

Diagnosis of the included patients were: adult scoliosis de novo in 79 cases (64.2%), degenerative spondylolisthesis (grade I/II according Meyerding classification) in 34 (27.6%), and isthmic spondylolisthesis (grade I/II according Meyerding classification) in 10 (8.2%). Demographical and clinical data are reported in Table 1.

Table 1. Enrolled patients data

Demographics	
N° of patients	123
Age	61.4 +/- 8.3
Sex	F 77, M 46
BMI	26.1, +/-1.7
Diabetes	18%
Smokers	36%
Diagnosis	
Degenerative Spondylolisthesis	34 (27.6%)
Adult Degenerative Scoliosis	79 (64.2%)
Isthmic Spondylolisthesis	10 (8.2%)
Instrumented level	n° 198
L1-2	6 (3%)
L2-3	56 (23%)
L3-4	97 (48.5%)
L4-5	39 (19.5%)
Cage material	
PEEK	51 (25.8%)
Titanium	147 (74.2%)
Cage Bone graft	
Attrax™	62 (31%)
ß tricalcium-phosphate	95 (43.5%)
Demineralized bone matrix	41 (20.5%)
Mean Follow Up	18.8+/- 1.1

3.2. Surgical Data

A total of 198 intersomatic cages were implanted, of which 147 (74.2%) made by titanium and 51 (25.8%) made by PEEK. The instrumentated segment was L1-L2 in 6 (3%) cases, L2-L3 in 56 (23%) cases, L3-L4 in 97 (48.5%), and L4-L5 in 39 (19.5%). One hundred and sixty (80%) cages were 10° lordotic, whereas 38 (20%) were flat. Attrax™ was used as graft filling material in 62 (31%) cages, ß tricalcium-phosphate in 95 (43.5%), and demineralized bone matrix in 41 (20.5%) cages. The mean ileal-psoas muscle retraction duration was 26 min (± 5.3, range 17–31) for each level treated. The mean intraoperative blood loss was 145.2 (±60.4, range 63–200) ml. Only two cases of adult scoliosis with long posterior instrumentation required blood transfusion (1 unit of concentrated blood cells). No intraoperative complications were observed. No cases of endplate violation were documented. Twelve (9.7%) cases of transient dysesthesia on the anterior surface of the thigh (10 ipsilateral to the surgical approach and 2 contralateral) were observed. Ten cases (8.1%) of postoperative paralytic ileus (spontaneously recovered) were recorded. The presence of abdominal wall twitching was observed in 5 (4%) patients. In 2 cases a superficial wound infection on posterior percutaneous access occurred. Postoperative complications did not require reoperation in any case.

3.3. Radiological Findings

According to the criteria for assessing fusion proposed by Berjano et al. [15], among the 198 level instrumented, we recorded 75% (149 cage) of segments with complete fusion (F), 19% (36 cages) of stable and probably fused (PF) segments, and 6% (13 cages) segments in pseudarthrosis (P). Pseudarthrosis occurred in 7 and 6 segments in where was implanted a titanium or PEEK cage, respectively. CS occurred in 13 (6.5%) cases. The spinopelvic parameters, measured preoperatively, immediately postoperatively and at last radiological follow-up, changed as follows:

- Lumbar Lordosis (LL) 39.9° (± 9.1), 51.8° (± 10.2), 46.7 (± 9.7 p = 0.002 between postoperative and 12 months follow up measurement);
- Sacral Slope (SS) 26 .5° (± 7.6), 31.2° (± 5.4), 29.3° (± 6.2; p = 0.317 between postoperative and 12 months follow up measurement);
- Pelvic Tilt (PT) 22.2° (± 3.9), 19.1° (± 5.1), 20.7° (± 6.2; p = 0.46 between postoperative and 12 months follow up measurement).
- No statistically significant differences were measured comparing PI modifications over the follow-up.

The mean disc angle of single level treated changed from 2.4° (± 0.9) preoperatively to 5.9 (± 1.7) immediately post operatively (p = 0.0217), then to 5.3 (± 1.9) 12 months after surgery (p= 0.876).

3.3. Clinical and Functional Outcomes

The VAS back improved from a pre-operative score of 7.3 (± 1.6) to a 12-months post-operative score of 3.1 (± 0.6) (p < 0.001) in patients completely fused, from 7.8 (± 1.1) to 3.6 (± 0.7) (p = 0.0032) in probably fused group, and from 8.2(± 1.2) to 5.1 (± 1.7) in patients with pseudarthrosis (p = 0.0074). The VAS back score of patients with pseudarthrosis was significatively higher than patients belonging to fused (p = 0.0013) and probably fused (p = 0.0062) groups. The ODI score improved from a pre-operative value of 48% (± 8.6) to a 12-months post-operative value of 25% (± 12.5) (p < 0.001) in patients completely fused, from 52% (± 10.3) to 28% (± 9.8) (p = 0.0049) in probably fused group, and from 56%(± 12.1) to 38% (± 13.8) in patients with pseudarthrosis (p = 0.0037). The ODI score of patients with pseudarthrosis was significatively higher than patients belonging to fused (p = 0.003) and probably fused (p = 0.007) groups.

3.4. Subgroups Analysis

Stratifying the enrolled patients in three groups (F, PF, P) we recorded a higher CS rate in group P (61.5%) compared with group PF (8.3%) and group F (1.3%). Concerning LL, the group P recorded the major loss of correction (49.1° ± 7.3 vs 39.2 ± 6.2, p= 0.0327) compared with the group PF and the group F between postoperative and 12 months follow up measurement.

4. Discussion

4.1. Background and Summary of Evidence

Although LLIF along with percutaneous PTSF represents a widespread and widely used procedure, there are still few papers in the literature that analyse and quantify the interbody fusion rate after these procedures [11, 13, 15, 16-20]. The gold standard radiological exam for the evaluation of fusion rate remains the fine cut CT scan with multiplanar reconstructions [11]. The stimmed fusion rate assessed by CT scan, range between 78 and 93% in the literature [11, 13, 15, 16-20].

Rodgers et al. [13], in a prospective study, analysed clinical results and the fusion rate of 66 patients (for a total of 88 segments) after XLIF procedures, using Thin-slice (1 mm) CT scans with sagittal reconstructions. They found a solid fusion (presence of complete or incomplete bone bridge between two contiguous vertebral endplate) in 96.6% of the treated levels, 12 months after surgery.

Berjano et al. [15] in a retrospective study, investigated the fusion rate after 12 months of follow up, in 53 patients treated with LLIF, using CT scan with coronal and sagittal reconstructions. They found a complete fusion in 87.1% of patients, a probably fusion in 10.2%, and pseudarthrosis in 2.6% of patients. The authors sustained that there was no statistically significant difference in terms of clinical and functional results between patients declared fused and patients with incomplete fusion or pseudarthrosis [15].

Malham and colleagues [16] in a retrospective study, analyzed the fusion rate after 12 months of follow up in 30 patients treated with LLIF procedure. The authors reported a fusion rate as high as 85%, evaluating HD CT coronal views images. The authors sustained that patients with supplementary internal fixation achieved a higher fusion rate, compared to those with stand alone cages. However, going through data, this difference seems to be not statistically significant. Furthermore, in their investigation the authors did not use an univocal method for evaluating fusion.

Rodgers et al., [17] in a prospective study, analysed the fusion rate following LLIF procedure in 44 patients, using CT scan imaging at 12 months after surgery. They used the modified Bridwell grading system [21] to quantify the fusion rate, and a different scale to describe the volume of bone present in the disc space. The authors observed a radiographic fusion in 41 of 44 treated levels (93.2%).

Ozgur et al., [18] in a retrospective chart review of prospectively collected clinical and radiographic data, measured outcomes of 62 patients who underwent LLIF for degenerative conditions, including degenerative disk disease, spondylolisthesis, scoliosis, and stenosis. In the radiographic outcomes, the authors included the identification of successful arthrodesis, evaluated using post-operative plain radiographs, obtained two years after surgery. Ozgur defined as fusion the presence of a bridging trabecular bone between the 2 treated vertebrae, along with the lack of lucencies on plain radiographs [18]. The authors observed that fusion was achieved in 91% of patients. Only one patient with pseudarthrosis required revision surgery. The authors concluded that there were no statistical differences in fusion rates based on diagnosis.

Parker et al. [19] in a prospective study evaluated the radiologic and clinical outcome of 135 consecutive patients who underwent lateral lumbar interbody fusion. The cages were filled with β- calcium triphosphate or recombinant Human Bone Morphogenetic Protein (rhBMP-2). They used a high-definition CT scans with multiplanar reconstruction performed 24 months after surgery. Fusion was defined as the presence of bridging interbody trabecular bone, according Williams et al. definition [22]. The authors concluded that the fusion rate was significantly higher for rhBMP-2 with 96% compared to 80% for β-TCP. However, stratifying the treated patients into those with a standalone cage and those with supplemental posterior instrumentation, there was no significant difference between instrumented fusion rates between β-TCP and rhBMP-2. While for standalone patients there was a significant difference with higher fusion rates in the rhBMP-2 group.

Dakwar et al. [20] retrospectively reviewed a prospectively acquired database of all patients with adult thoracolumbar degenerative deformity treated with LLIF. They analyzed the fusion rate in 25 patients using CT scan with multiplanar reconstruction and flexion-extension radiographs performed 6 months after surgery. They found the evidence of radiographic fusion in the 80% of the treated patients. However, the authors did not describe any univocal method for fusion rate assessment.

Gao et al., [23] in a retrospective study, analyzed the clinical and radiological outcomes of 93 patients following LLIF procedure. They divided the patients according the bone graft materials into: allogeneic bone groups (group A), rhBMP-2 + allogenic bone (group B), and autologous bone marrow + allogeneic bone (group C). The fusion rate was evaluated with a using the Williams et al. method [22] and the Tohmeh et al. [24] grading to evaluate the rate of intervertebral fusion. The fusion rate in group A was 71.0%, in group B 93.8%, while in the group C was 86.7%

Tohmeh et al. [24] in a prospective study, analyzed clinical and radiological results in a cohort of 40 patients who underwent LLIF procedure, followed by PTSF using CT scan images performed 12 months after surgery. They found a complete fusion in 90.2% of the treated levels, while the remaining 9.8% of treated patients were partially consolidated and progressing towards fusion.

Umebayashi and colleagues [25] reported their experience on LLIF using porous hydroxyapatite/collagen composite as grafts within the cages. The authors observed a fusion rate of 81%.

Proietti et al. [11] in a retrospective radiological study evaluated the clinical and radiological outcomes in a homogenous cohort of 74 patients affected by degenerative spondylolisthesis who underwent LLIF procedures following by percutaneous PTSF. The authors proposed a new topographical classification using fine cut CT scan images obtained 12 months after surgery. They found the presence of intervertebral BB in 78.3% of the treated patients.

Although the fusion rate is an increasingly used radiological parameter to evaluate the solidity of interbody fusion, non-homogeneous methods for evaluating a segment as fused have been reported and a consensus on the way for assessing this outcome is still missing.

4.2. Fusion Rate and Classification System

In the past two decades, many efforts have been made to define, classify and identify interbody fusion. Many authors in Literature, with this aim, tried to devise radiological or functional classifications. In this paragraph, the purpose of the authors was to describe the most important and adopted classifications for interbody fusion.

4.2.1. Evaluation of the Fusion Rate, and Related Radiological Techniques

For many years, before the advent of modern radiological imaging techniques such as CT scans, dynamic lateral flexion and extension radiographs were considered as gold standard method to evaluate the presence and the progression of an interbody fusion [22, 26]. However, this technique presented a high intra- and interobserver variability. The quality of the images, often inadequate, and the presence of artifacts due to metallic material, make difficult to evaluate interbody fusion. Furthermore, it is frequently not possible to distinguish the presence of newly formed bone from the bone-like graft material, placed into the fusion device and around the implant in to the disc space, especially when using autologous bone. [27]. Moreover, both static and dynamic radiographs, seems to overestimate the anterior interbody fusion rate [28].

Since its appearance, CT scan rapidly became the most used radiological technique in the evaluation of interbody fusion. This technique allows to obtain high quality images with reconstructions in the coronal and sagittal planes, resulting in a much more accurate assessment of interbody fusion [29].

The presence of BB and new bone formation within or adjacent to the fusion device became visible on CT images typically 3 months after surgery and usually progresses for up to 18 –24 months. BB formation is easily evaluated on the coronal and sagittal reconstructions, and may represent a pathognomonic sign of interbody fusion [22].

Based on CT images many interbody fusion classification were made.

4.2.2. Bridwell's Classification

This classification in one of the most used to identify a solid fusion of a vertebral segment. Originally, Bridwell et al. [21] designed their classifications on plain radiographs, however, nowadays the same concept could be used on CT images.

The authors performed two classification systems:

- The anterior fusion grade: this classification regard the anterior elements and properly the interbody fusion. The authors identified four grade of fusion, divided as follow: Grade I, fusion of the two vertebral endplate with remodelling of the graft and trabeculae formation; Grade II, Graft intact, no fully incorporated and remodelled, no presence of lucency; Grade III, Graft intact, presence of a definite lucency at the top or at the bottom of the graft; Grade IV, non fused, resorbtion and collapse of the graft.
- The posterior fusion grade. This classification regards the posterior elements, specifically zygapophyseal joints and trasverse processes. The authors identified four grade of fusion, divided as follow: Grade I, solid trabeculated trasverse process and bilaterally fusion of facet joints; Grade II, presence of thick fusion mass monolaterally; Grade III; Suspected lucency or defect in fusion mass; Grade IV, resorption of the graft material and fatigue of the instrumentation.

These classifications are generic for segmental vertebral fusion and non specially designed for LLIF procedure.

4.2.3. Tan's Classification

This classification was designed for the evaluation of a solid fusion after anterior column reconstruction of the thoracolumbar spine with a structural allograft [28]. However, some authors suggested to extend the use of this bony fusion assessment method based on high-speed spiral CT imaging to other procedures [15]. Tan et al. [28] defined 4 degree of fusion, described as follows:

- Grade I, complete fusion: there was a cortical union of the allograft and central trabecular continuity.
- Grade II, partial fusion: when the cortical union of the structural allograft had a partial trabecular incorporation.
- Grade III, unipolar pseudarthrosis: denotes superior or inferior cortical non-union of the central allograft with partial trabecular discontinuity centrally
- Grade IV, bipolar pseudarthrosis: suggests both superior and inferior cortical non-union with a complete lack of central trabecular continuity.

4.2.4. Tohmeh's Classification

This classification is based on CT images with sagittal and coronal reconstructions, obtained from patients who underwent to LLIF procedure and PTSF. The authors examine only the anterior elements for the assessment of interbody fusion. The classification consists in three degree, organized as follows:

- Grade I, complete fusion with complete ossification with some component of endplate involvement;
- Grade II, incomplete/progressing fusion with ossification in cage that abuts one or both endplates without evidence of endplate involvement or continuous bridging bone;
- Grade III, indeterminate; clear lucencies at endplates with or without ossification in the cage.

Although this classification is very simple and reproducible, it has been not widely adopted, and is getting even more obsolete.

4.2.5. Berjano's Classification

This CT images based classification appears very similar to the Tohmeh's one. The authors [15] identified 3 grade of fusion, according to the following criteria:

- Grade I, Fusion (F), when a bone bridge is recognized in the interbody space, connecting the lower endplate of the cranial vertebra to the upper endplate of the caudal vertebra;
- Grade II, Stable/probably fused (PF) when partial radiolucency was observed at only one interface of the graft-endplate contact but no bone resorption was present around the cage or screws;
- Grade III, Pseudarthrosis (P) when no graft material was visible in the cage, complete radiolucency was seen at both interfaces, or when radiolucency was observed in one interface with additional bone resorption surrounding the cage or the screws.

4.2.6. Proietti's Classification

This classification seems to be different from the aforementioned ones, since it tries to evaluate not only the fusion status of an instrumented vertebral segment, but also the residual mobility grade. Furthermore, it is specifically designed for evaluating fusion after LLIF, and the presence of BB is also described in a topographical way, according to the surgical technique and cages shape and characteristics. [11], according Williams's definition [22] inside and outside the cage. They detected seven type of BB formation, described as follows:

Type I: no bone bridges (no fusion).
Type II: bone bridges inside one of the two internal spaces of the cage.
Type III: bone bridges in both internal spaces of the cage.
Type IV: bone bridges inside one of the two internal spaces of the cage and on one side.
Type V: bone bridges inside one of the two internal spaces of the cage and on both sides.
Type VI: complete fusion of the inside the cage, and on and on one side.
Type VII: complete fusion of the inside the cage, and on both sides.

Only the type I was considered non fused.

The authors evalued also the posterior elements fusion status, according to Pathria et al. classification [30, 31] modified as follows:

- Grade 0, normal facet joints;
- Grade I, narrowing joint rim, small osteophyte or mild hypertrophy of the articular process;
- Grade II, narrowing joint rim with mild subarticular bone erosions;
- Grade III, ankylosis.

The segments with Pathria Grade III, thus ankylotic degeneration of the zygapophyseal joints, were considered posteriorly fused, therefore immobilized.

Combining the two classifications the authors described 3 grade of fusion as follows:

- Non-fusion: no evidence of BB between the two vertebral endplates or posterior facet joints ankylosis (Pathria grade ranging from 0 to II);
- Partial fusion: either interbody BB or facet joints ankylotic degeneration (Patria grade III);
- Circumferential fusion: both anterior BB and ankylotic facet joints.

Although this classification may result as more complex when firstly approaching it, it is the only one evaluating the entire vertebral segment (anterior and posterior elements) and the immobilization grade, which has to be considered as the real goal in spinal fusion surgeries. In fact, non-residual immobilization is the result of a solid instrumentation, and it provide less fatigue on the system, which is not exposed to load-dependent movements, thus resulting in lower chances for its mechanical failure.

4.3. Bone Graft Material

The clinical and radiologic success of lumbar spine fusion surgery depends on many factors. Certainly, the presence of a solid bone fusion represents one of the most relevant. [32]. Multiple variables could influence the bony fusion after lumbar fusion surgeries, such as the presence of bone-forming cells that could drive osteogenesis process, bioactive osteoinductive growth factors, osteoconductive scaffold that provides structural support for new bone formation, represented by graft material and cage structure [33].

Different graft materials used for cage filling were described in the Literature. The autologous bone grafts, already demonstrated as effective in different skeletal segments [13, 14, 34], should be considered as the first choice. However, due to the comorbidity of the donor site and the increasing use of minimally invasive techniques, with particular attention to aesthetic results [35], it is increasingly difficult to take autologous bone grafts. A valid alternative could be represented by compatible heterologous bone graft, however, the scarce availability and the high prices make this solution not very usable [36]. Recently, even more spinal surgeons successfully reported the use of synthetic or semi-synthetic bone substitutes, such as β-TCP, rhBMP-2, porous hydroxyapatite/collagen composite, Attrax™ (Nuvasive Inc., San Diego, CA, USA), Nanostim™ (Medtronic, Memphis, TN, USA), as bone graft during spinal fusion procedures [11, 13-20, 24,25]. Most authors reported no significant differences regarding the fusion rate by stratifying patients by the type of graft used to fill the cage [15-18, 24-25].

Relatively few reports observed a superiority of rhBMP-2 over other graft materials [19, 23]. Unfortunately, the use of rhBMP-2 as grafting material in spinal surgery showed a high rate of complications. Mroz et al. [37], in a review article analysed the complications rate following BMP use in spinal surgery, reporting a 44% of resorption/osteolysis, 25% of graft subsidence, 8% of ectopic bone growth, 27% of cage migration, 29% incidence of new onset radiculitis, and an inflammatory response to the collagen carrier in 29% of patients. In our opinion, the choice of graft material had a quiet marginal role in influencing the fusion rate. A good primary stability that leads to a secondary bony fusion could be the result to be pursued, eventually influencing the fusion rate. However, a clear scientific evidence is still missing. Future properly designed clinical trials with will better clarify this topic.

4.4. Our Experience

Our series represents one of the largest presented in the international medical literature. According to Proietti et al. [11], in our series the fusion rate is lower than the average from the literature. Although three different types of graft materials were used, no statistically significant difference was found in fusion rate. Conversely, a strong correlation was found between CS and pseudarthrosis. In fact, over than 65% of the patients belonging to the P group had a subsidence of the cage. Furthermore, a greater LL loss, compared to group F and group PF, was found in patients belonging to group P. Therefore, the presence of pseudarthrosis, of CS and LL loss seem to be the variables that most affect the clinical outcome in patients with ASD who underwent LLIF and percutaneous PTSF.

Nevertheless, these informations need to be carefully interpretated, according to the non-negligible limitations of the present study: this is a retrospectively investigation, it lacks a controll group, an the relatively small number of patients may affect level of evidence.

CONCLUSION

The evaluation of fusion rate after LLIF represents a current and interesting topic. CT imaging, with fine-cut axial and multiplanar reconstructions, has to be considered as the gold standard to assess the fusion status after spinal fusion procedures. Although many classifications were designed to assess the interbody fusion rate following LLIF, none was validated on a large number of patients.

While many studies focused their attention on radiographic aspects, due to the low number of cases of pseudarthrosis, only few papers assessed the correlation between clinical outcomes and the fusion rate. However, the loss of lumbar lordosis correction, the presence of pseudartrosis, and the accorrence of cage subsidence seem to be related to a worst clinical outcome.

No graft material used to fill the cages, autologus, heterologus, sintetic and semi-sintetic, proved to be superior to the others and capable of determining a higher fusion rate.

No statistically significant difference was found in the literature on the difference in fusion rate based on the cage material (PEEK, titanium or carbon fiber)

However, the fusion rate remains as high as > 78%, thus higher than other posterior lumbar fusion techniques.

REFERENCES

[1] Barone G, Scaramuzzo L, Zagra A, Giudici F, Perna A, Proietti L. (2017) Adult spinal deformity: effectiveness of interbody lordotic cages to restore disc angle and spino-pelvic parameters through completely mini-invasive trans-psoas and hybrid approach. *Eur Spine J.* 26(Suppl 4):457-463. doi:10.1007/s00586-017-5136-1.

[2] Tamburrelli FC, Meluzio MC, Burrofato A, Perna A, Proietti L. (2018) Minimally invasive surgery procedure in isthmic spondylolisthesis. *Eur Spine J.* 27(Suppl 2):237-243. doi:10.1007/s00586-018-5627-8.

[3] Ricciardi L, Stifano V, Proietti L, et al. (2018) Intraoperative and Postoperative Segmental Lordosis Mismatch: Analysis of 3 Fusion Techniques. *World Neurosurg.* 115:e659-e663. doi:10.1016/j.wneu.2018.04.126.

[4] Mokawem M, Katzouraki G, Harman CL, Lee R. (2019) Lumbar interbody fusion rates with 3D-printed lamellar titanium cages using a silicate-substituted calcium phosphate bone graft. *J Clin Neurosci.* 68:134-139. doi:10.1016/j.jocn.2019.07.011.

[5] Tamburrelli FC, Perna A, Proietti L, Zirio G, Santagada DA, Genitiempo M. (2019) The Feasibility of Long-Segment Fluoroscopy-guided Percutaneous Thoracic Spine Pedicle Screw Fixation, and the Outcome at Two-year Follow-up. *Malays Orthop J.* 13(3):39-44. doi:10.5704/MOJ.1911.007.

[6] Watkins R 4th, Watkins R 3rd, Hanna R. Non-union rate with stand-alone lateral lumbar interbody fusion. *Medicine* (Baltimore). 2014;93(29):e275. doi:10.1097/MD.0000000000000275.

[7] Logroscino CA, Tamburrelli FC, Scaramuzzo L, Schirò GR, Sessa S, Proietti L. (2012) Transdiscal L5-S1 screws for the treatment of adult spondylolisthesis. *Eur Spine J.* 21 (Suppl 1):S128-S133. doi:10.1007/s00586-012-2229-8.

[8] Kumagai H, Abe T, Koda M, et al. (2019) Unidirectional porous β-tricalcium phosphate induces bony fusion in lateral lumbar interbody fusion. *J Clin Neurosci.* 59:232-235. doi:10.1016/j.jocn.2018.09.004.

[9] Takeuchi M, Kamiya M, Wakao N, Hirasawa A, Kawanami K, Osuka K, et al. (2015) Large volume inside the cage leading incomplete interbody bone fusion and residual back pain after posterior lumbar interbody fusion. *Neurosurg Rev* 38(3):573–8.

[10] McAfee PC, Boden SD, Brantigan JW, et al. Symposium: a critical discrepancy-a criteria of successful arthrodesis following interbody spinal fusions. (2001) *Spine* (Phila Pa 1976). 26(3):320-334. doi:10.1097/00007632-200102010-00020.

[11] Proietti L, Perna A, Ricciardi L, et al. (2020) Radiological evaluation of fusion patterns after lateral lumbar interbody fusion: institutional case series. *Radiol Med;*10.1007/s11547-020-01252-5. doi:10.1007/s11547-020-01252-5.

[12] McAfee PC, Boden SD, Brantigan JW et al. (2001) Symposium: a critical discrepancy-a criteria of successful arthrodesis following interbody spinal fusions. *Spine* 26:320–334.

[13] Rodgers WB, Gerber EJ, Patterson JR (2010) Fusion after mini- mally disruptive anterior lumbar interbody fusion: analysis of extreme lateral interbody fusion by computed tomography. *SAS J* 4:63–66. https://doi.org/10.1016/j.esas.2010.03.001.

[14] Ozgur BM, Aryan HE, Pimenta L, Taylor WR (2006) Extreme lateral interbody fusion (XLIF): a novel surgical technique for anterior lumbar interbody fusion. *Spine J* 6:435–443. https://doi.org/10.1016/j.spinee.2005.08.012.

[15] Berjano P, Langella F, Damilano M et al. (2015) Fusion rate following extreme lateral lumbar interbody fusion. *Eur Spine J* 24(Suppl 3):369–371. https://doi.org/10.1007/s00586-015-3929-7.

[16] Malham GM, Ellis NJ, Parker RM, Seex KA (2012) Clinical outcome and fusion rates after the first 30 extreme lat- eral interbody fusions. *Sci World J* 2012:246989. https://doi.org/10.1100/2012/246989.

[17] Rodgers WB, Gerber EJ, Rodgers JA. (2012) Clinical and radiographic outcomes of 4 extreme lateral approach to interbody fusion with β-tricalcium phosphate and 5 hydroxyapatite composite for lumbar degenerative conditions. *Int J Spine Surg.* 6:24-28..

[18] Ozgur BM, Agarwal V, Nail E, Pimenta L. (2010) Two-year clinical and radiographic success of minimally invasive lateral transpsoas approach for the treatment of degenerative lumbar conditions. *SAS J.;* 4(2):41-46. Published 2010 Jun 1. doi:10.1016/j.esas.2010.03.005.

[19] Parker RM, Malham GM. (2017) Comparison of a calcium phosphate bone substitute with recombinant human bone morphogenetic protein-2: a prospective study of fusion rates, clinical outcomes and complications with 24-month follow-up. *Eur Spine J.* 26(3):754-763. doi:10.1007/s00586-016-4927-0.

[20] Dakwar E, Cardona RF, Smith DA, Uribe JS. (2010) Early outcomes and safety of the minimally invasive, lateral retroperitoneal transpsoas approach for adult degenerative scoliosis. *Neurosurg Focus;* 28(3):E8. doi:10.3171/2010.1.FOCUS09282.

[21] Bridwell KH, Lenke G, McEnery KW, Baldus C, Blanke K. (1995) Anterior fresh frozen structural allografts in the thoracic and lumbar spine. Do they work if combined with posterior fusion and instrumentation in adult patients with kyphosis or anterior column defects? *Spine* (Phila Pa 1976); 20:1410–8.

[22] Williams AL, Gornet MF, Burkus JK (2005) CT evaluation of lumbar interbody fusion: current concepts. *AJNR Am J Neuroradiol* 26:2057-2066.

[23] Gao Y, Li J, Cui H, et al. (2019) Comparison of intervertebral fusion rates of different bone graft materials in extreme lateral interbody fusion. *Medicine (Baltimore).*;98(44):e17685. doi:10.1097/MD. 0000000000017685.

[24] Tohmeh AG, Blake W, Mirna T, et al. (2012) Allograft cellular bone matrix in extreme lateral interbody fusion: preliminary radiographic and clinical outcomes. *Sci World J.* 2012:1–8.

[25] Umebayashi T, Ohta K, Mitsuyama T, Ohshima K, Kohno R, Kumano K. (2017) Fusion rate following lateral lumbar interbody fusion using porous hydroxyapatite/collagen composite at 1-year follow-up. *J Spine Res;* 8:1299 302.

[26] Blumenthal SL, Gill K. (1993) Can lumbar spine radiographs accurately determine fusion in post-operative patients? Correlation of routine radiographs with a second surgical look at lumbar fusions. *Spine;* 18:1186–1189.

[27] Schuler TC, Subach BR, Branch CL, et al. (2004) Segmental lumbar lordosis: manual versus computer-assisted measurement using seven different techniques. *J Spinal Disord Tech* 17:372–379.

[28] Tan G, Goss B, Thorpe P, Williams R (2007) CT-based classi- fication of long spinal allograft fusion. *Eur Spine J* 16(11):1875–1881.

[29] Rothman SLG, Glenn WV Jr. (1985) CT evaluation of interbody fusion. *Clin Orthop Rel Res;*193:47–56.

[30] Pathria M, Sartoris DJ, Resnick D (1987) Osteoarthritis of the facet joints: accuracy of oblique radiographic assessment. *Radiology* 164:227–230. https://doi.org/10.1148/radio logy.164.1.3588910.

[31] Proietti L, Scaramuzzo L, Schirò GR et al. (2015) Degenerative facet joint changes in lumbar percutaneous pedicle screw fixation without fusion. *Orthop Traumatol Surg Res 101*:375–379. https://doi.org/10.1016/j.otsr.2015.01.013.

[32] Djurasovic M, Glassman SD, Dimar JR, Howard JM, Bratcher KR, Carreon LY (2011) Does fusion status correlate with patient outcomes in lumbar spinal fusion? *Spine* 36:404–409.

[33] Lee YP, Pattnaik T, Garfin SR (2013) Biologic considerations in XLIF. In: Goodrich JA, Volcan IJ (eds) *Extreme lateral interbody* fusion

(XLIF), 2nd edn. Quality Medical Publishing Inc, St. Louis, pp 137–145.

[34] De Vitis R, Passiatore M, Perna A, Tulli A, Pagliei A, Taccardo G. (2019) Modified Matti-Russe technique using a "butterfly bone graft" for treatment of scaphoid non-union. *J Orthop.* 19:63-66. Published 2019 Nov 27. doi:10.1016/j.jor.2019.11.030.

[35] Ricciardi L, Sturiale CL, Pucci R, et al. (2019) Patient-Oriented Aesthetic Outcome after Lumbar Spine Surgery: A 1-Year Follow-Up Prospective Observational Study Comparing Minimally Invasive and Standard Open Procedures. *World Neurosurg.* 122:e1041-e1046. doi:10.1016/j.wneu.2018.10.208.

[36] Barbera G, Raponi I, Nocini R, Della Monaca M, Priore P, Valentini V. (2020) Secondary Rhinoplasty in Binder Syndrome: Considerations and Management of Complex Problem With Heterologous Bone Graft [published online ahead of print, 2020 Jul 17]. *J Craniofac Surg.;* 10.1097/SCS.0000000000006789. doi:10.1097/SCS.0000000000006789.

[37] Mroz TE, Wang JC, Hashimoto R, Norvell DC. (2010) Complications related to osteobiologics use in spine surgery: a systematic review. *Spine.* 35(9, suppl):S86–S104.

BIOGRAPHICAL SKETCH

Alessandro Ramieri, MD, PhD

Affiliation: Faculty of Pharmacy and Medicine, Dpt Orthopaedics and Traumatology. University, "La Sapienza" of Rome, Italy

Education: Rome University "La Sapienza", Eurospine, AO Spine

Research and Professional Experience:

July 1995 Graduate Medicine and Surgery Sapienza Rome University
July 1996-July1997 Medical Officer Italian Army

Nov 2002-present	Post-graduate Degree in Orthopaedics and Traumatology, Sapienza Rome University
May 2011	PhD Pathophysiology and Muscle-Skeletal Disorders, Sapienza Rome University
May 2014-present	Research Fellow and Teacher, Sapienza Rome University
Nov 2011	European Spine Course Diploma (Budapest session)
Feb 2014	Eurospine TFR Course Diploma (Dublin)
May 2000	GIS-Italian Spine Society Member (Ordinary)
Apr 2014-present	AOSPINE Member (Silver)
Apr 2003- Mar 2004	spinal surgeon S. Pertini Rome Hospital
Gen 2005-Apr 2018	orthopaedic consultant Sapienza Polo Pontino ICOT, Latina
Gen 2005-present	orthopaedic consultant Don Gnocchi Onlus Foundation, Milan
Gen 2011-present	orthopaedic consultant Capodarco Onlus Foundation, Rome
Apr 2020-present	Resercher and Professor, University La Sapienza, Rome Italy

Scholastic screening for AIS prevention in 2002; Several projects in the field of spinal diseases for the Italian Ministry of Health from 2010 to 2015; Teacher and tutor in Master Courses on Mininvasive Techniques in Spinal Pathologies, S. Andrea Hosp, Sapienza University, Rome Italy; Tutor in the AOSpine course "Thoracolumbar Spine Stabilization", Rome 2014; Teacher in "Neurophysiopathological Techniques", MIPAD Lazio, Sapienza Rome University, 2007-08.

Editorial Board Member for WJO-*World Journal of Orthopaedics*; Editorial Board Member for JSM-Neurosurgery and Spine; Reviewer for *World Journal of Orthopedics*, *J. Neuroscience in Rural Practice*, *Neurosurgical Review*, *J Neurology Neurosugery and Psychiatry*, *Annals of case report*, *Annals of Orthopaedics*, *Journal of Pain Research*, *Scientific Journal of Neurology and Neurosurgery; Orth. Research and Review* (Dove Press)

Professional Appointments: AO International Validation Group on "AO Spine Subaxial Fractures classification system international validation study" e "AO Spine Sacral classification system validation study"

Honors:

- 1995 Tagliapietra Award, Sinch-Italian Neurosurgery Society;
- 2000 GIS Scholarship, GIS Italian Spine Society

Publications for the Last Three Years:

1. Ramieri Alessandro, Giorgio Ippolito, Umberto Prencipe, Giovanni Corsini, Maurizio Domenicucci, Giuseppe Costanzo (2020): Chapter 34. Osteolytic metastases of the thoracolumbar spine: the role of the vertebroplasty and kyphoplasty. In: Landi A, Gregori F, Delfini R: *Spinal cord and spinal column tumors.* Nova Science Publishers, Inc., Hauppauge NY, 11788 USA, ISBN: 978-1-53616-474-9.
2. Miscusi M, Ramieri A, Forcato S, Trungu S, Domenicucci M, Costanzo G, Raco A (2020): Chapter 33: Minimally Invasive Spinal Surgery (MISS) for Neurological Metastases of the Thoracic and Lumbar Spine. In: Landi A, Gregori F, Delfini R: *Spinal cord and spinal column tumors.* Nova Science Publishers, Inc., Hauppauge NY, 11788 USA, ISBN: 978-1-53616-474-9.
3. Ramieri A, Domenicucci M, Corsini G, Campopiano G, Miscusi M (2017). Functional anatomy e biomechanics of the axial and subaxial cervical spine. In: Delfini R, Landi A. *Cervical Spine Surgery*, ROME CIC International Editions, ISBN: 8893890054.
4. Ramieri A, Polli FM, Manauzzi E, Meloncelli S, Costanzo G (2017). Posterior cervical interfacet fixation : DTRAX® system. In: Delfini R, Landi A, *Cervical Spine Surgery.* ROME CIC International Editions, ISBN: 8893890054.
5. Domenicucci M, C Mancarella, G Santoro, DE Dugoni, A Ramieri. Spinal epidural hematomas: personal experience and literature

review of more than 1000 cases *Journal of Neurosurgery: Spine* 27 (2), 198-208, 2017.
6. Miscusi M, A Ramieri, S Forcato, M Giuffrè, S Trungu, M Cimatti, A Pesce. Comparison of pure lateral and oblique lateral inter-body fusion for treatment of lumbar degenerative disk disease: a multicentric cohort study. *European Spine Journal* 27 (2), 222-228, 2018.
7. Miscusi M, S Trungu, S Forcato, A Ramieri, FM Polli, A Raco. Long-term clinical outcomes and quality of life in elderly patients treated with interspinous devices for lumbar spinal stenosis. *Journal of Neurological Surgery Part A: Central European Neurosurgery* 79, 139-144, 2018.
8. Ramieri A, M Miscusi, M Domenicucci, A Raco, G Costanzo. Surgical management of coronal and sagittal imbalance of the spine without PSO: a multicentric cohort study on compensated adult degenerative deformities. *European Spine Journal* 26 (4), 442-449, 2017.
9. Ramieri A, D Marruzzo, P Missori, M Miscusi, R Tarantino, Lumbar ganglion cyst: Nosology, surgical management and proposal of a new classification based on 34 personal cases and literature review. M Domenicucci, *World Journal of Orthopedics* 8 (9), 697, 2017.
10. Santoro G, A Ramieri, V Chiarella, M Vigliotta, M Domenicucci. Thoraco-lumbar fractures with blunt traumatic aortic injury in adult patients: correlations and management. *European Spine Journal* 27 (2), 248-257, 2018.
11. Miscusi M., Serrao M., Conte C., Ippolito G., Marinozzi F., Bini F., Troise S., Forcato S., Trungu S., Ramieri A., Pierelli F., Raco A. (2019). Spatial and temporal characteristics of the spine muscles activation during walking in patients with lumbar instability due to degenerative lumbar disk disease: Evaluation in pre-surgical setting. *Human Movement Science,* vol. 66, p. 371-382, ISSN: 0167-9457, doi: 10.1016/j.humov.2019.05.013.

12. Chiarella V, A Ramieri, M Giugliano, M Domenicucci Rapid spontaneous resolution of lumbar ganglion cysts: A case report. *World Journal of Orthopedics* 11 (1): 68-75, 2020.
13. Miscusi Massimo, Alessandro Ramieri, Stefano Forcato, Sokol Trungu, Alessandro Pesce, Pietro Familiari, Giuseppe Costanzo, Antonino Raco (2019): Global Spine Congress, Toronto: Comparison of Clinical Outome and Spinopelvic Parameters Modifications Between Minimally Invasive and Conventional Open Posterior Lumbar Interbody Fusion for Treatment of High- Grade L5-S1 Isthmic Spondylolisthesis. *Global Spine Journal,* Vol. 9(2S) 2S-187S. The Author(s) 2019 Article reuse guidelines: sagepub.com/journals-permissions DOI: 10.1177/21925682 19839730 journals.sagepub.com/home/gsj.
14. Ramieri Alessandro, Stefano Forcato, Sokol Trungu, Alessandro Pesce, Pietro Familiari, Massimo Miscusi, Giuseppe Costanzo, Antonino Raco (2019): Global Spine Congress, Toronto: Lateral Lumbar Inter-Body Fusion in Lumbar Adult Deformities: Fusion Rate and Results. *Global Spine Journal,* Vol. 9(2S) 2S-187S. The Author(s) 2019 Article reuse guidelines: sagepub.com/journals-permissions DOI: 10.1177/2192568219839730 journals.sagepub.com/home/gsj.
15. Domenicucci Maurizio, Alessandro Ramieri (2018): Global Spine Congress, Singapore: Lumbar Ganglion Cyst: Nosology, Surgical Management and Proposal of a New Classification Based on 34 Personal Cases and Literature Review. *Global Spine Journal,* Vol. 8(1S) 2S-173S. The Author(s) 2018 Reprints and permission: sagepub.com/journals Permissions.nav DOI: 10.1177/219256821 8771030 journals.sagepub.com/home/gsj.
16. Ramieri Alessandro, Giuseppe Costanzo, Massimo Miscusi, Antonino Raco (2018): Restoring Lumbar Lordosis and Balance of the Spine without Pso or Vcr: Multicentric Experience On A Cohort Of 50 Consecutive Adult Degenerative Kyphoscoliosis. *Global Spine Journal,* Vol. 8(1S) 174S-374S The Author(s) 2018 Reprints and permission: sagepub.com/journalsPermissions.nav DOI:

10.1177/2192568218771072journals.sagepub.com/home/gsj.
17. Ramieri Alessandro, Giuseppe Costanzo (2018): FMwand in Posterior and Lateral Surgery for Spinal Deformities: Clinical and Radiological Study. *Global Spine Journal,* Vol. 8(1S) 174S-374S. The Author(s) 2018 Reprints and permission: sagepub.com/journals Permissions.nav DOI: 10.1177/2192568218771072 journals.sagepub.com/home/gsj.
18. Santoro Giorgio, Alessandro Ramieri, Maurizio Domenicucci: Global Spine Congress, Singapore: Thoraco-Lumbar Fractures With Traumatic Aortic Injury (TAI) in Adult Patients: Classification and Management. *Global Spine Journal* 2018, Vol. 8(1S) 2S-173S. The Author(s) 2018 Reprints and permission: sagepub.com/journals Permissions.nav DOI: 10.1177/2192568218771030.
19. Miscusi Massimo, Stefano Forcato, Filippo Maria Polli, Alessandro Ramieri, Marco Cimatti, Giuseppe Costanzo, Antonino Raco (2017): Global Spine Congress, Milano: Pure Lateral and Oblique Lateral Inter-body Fusion for Treatment of Lumbar Degenerative Disk Disease: Comparison of Two Different Techniques. *Global Spine Journal,* Vol. 7(2S) 2S-189S. The Author(s) 2017 Reprints and permission: sagepub.com/journals Permissions.nav DOI: 10.1177/2192568217708577 journals.sagepub.com/home/gsj.
20. Ramieri Alessandro, Massimo Miscusi, Filippo Maria Polli, Giuseppe Costanzo (2017): Global Spine Congress, Milano: Safety and Efficacy of Multilevel XLIFs Approaching the Convex Side of Adult Scoliosis above 30 Degrees. *Global Spine Journal,* Vol. 7(2S) 2S-189S. The Author(s) 2017 Reprints and permission: sagepub.com/journalsPermissions.nav. DOI: 10.1177/219256821 7708577 journals.sagepub.com/home/gsj.
21. Trongu Sokol, Massimo Miscusi, Luca Ricciardi, Stefano Forcato, Alessandro Ramieri, Antonino Raco. The ante-psoas approach (ATP) for interbody fusion at the L5-S1 segment: clinical and radiological outcomes [FOCUS20-335R1]. *J Neurosurgical Focus* (in press).

In: The Fundamentals of Spine Surgery
Editor: Tim Bachmeier

ISBN: 978-1-53618-570-6
© 2020 Nova Science Publishers, Inc.

Chapter 3

POSTERIOR FUSION IN DEGENERATIVE SPONDYLOLISTHESIS: THE ROLE OF THE MINIMALLY INVASIVE TRANSFORAMINAL APPROACH (MI-TLIF)

Alessandro Ramieri[*], *MD, PhD, Giorgio Rossi, MD, Omar Alshafeei, MD, Vincenzo Barci, MD and Giuseppe Costanzo, MD*
Faculty of Pharmacy and Medicine,
Department of Orthopedics and Traumatology,
University of "La Sapienza," Rome, Italy

ABSTRACT

There are numerous surgical options for patients with LDS (Lumbar Degenerative Spondylolisthesis). The operations are chosen accordingly to the surgeon's experience and his/her personal conduct and can be performed in an open or minimally invasive way. "What type of surgery" argument is still highly controversial and debated.

---

[*] Corresponding Author's E-mail: alexramieri@libero.it.

To date, a paucity of literature exists to evaluate safety and effectiveness of MI-TLIF (Minimally Invasive - Transforaminal Lumbar Interbody Fusion) in the treatment of LDS. The purpose of this paper is to show, in detail, the steps and technical procedures of this operation, as well as evaluating its short and long-term outcomes.

MI-TLIF, combined with Percutaneous Placement of Pedicle Screws and Rods, was performed in a cohort of 23 patients with LDS. In each patient, the level of anterolisthesis and the presence of a lumbar stenosis and/or herniated disc were verified. Operative data (operative time, estimated blood loss), length of hospitalization and complications were assessed. In the pre-operative and in the FUP (follow-up), VAS (Visual Analogue Scale) and ODI (Oswestry Disability Index) were calculated. In the FUP Radiographic check, MacNab score and Patient Satisfaction were also evaluated.

The total mean operative time was 170 ± 22.3 minutes and the mean blood loss was 205 ± 38.2 ml. The mean duration of hospitalization was 5 ± 1.6 days. No patient needed transfusion and none had infections. The total acquired neurological deficit rate was 13%. In the pre-operative and in the FUP, registered scores were compared using t-test. Statistically significant differences emerged in the VAS back ($p = 0.045$), in the VAS leg ($p = 0.018$) and in the ODI ($p = 0.013$). Furthermore, in the FUP the Radiographic check showed no implant problems and MacNab criteria had a good outcome in 78.3% of the patients. Eighteen patients would undergo this surgical operation again.

MI-TLIF may provide effective short and long term clinical-functional improvements in patients with LDS. Minimally invasive surgery guarantees a minimized tissue disruption and decreases the length of hospitalization and functional recovery times. Despite the possible post-operative root suffering, the technique can be considered safe and effective as shown in more than 80% of our patients.

Keywords: Lumbar Degenerative Spondylolisthesis (LDS), Minimally Invasive - Transforaminal Lumbar Interbody Fusion (MI-TLIF), percutaneous pedicle screw fixation

1. INTRODUCTION

1.1. Lumbar Degenerative Spondylolisthesis

Spondylolisthesis, from "spondylo" (vertebra) and "listhesis" (sliding), is the displacement of one vertebra compared to another. It can occur anteriorly (anterolisthesis), posteriorly (retrolisthesis) or laterally (laterolisthesis or lateral translation). The slippage of the vertebral body, compared to the adjacent one, generates a subluxation between the articular heads leading to a condition of vertebral instability.

Spondylolisthesis can be degenerative, dysplastic/congenital, traumatic or post-surgical/iatrogenic, and occurs most commonly in the lower lumbar spine.

The NASS (North American Spine Society) has defined LDS (Lumbar Degenerative Spondylolisthesis) as an acquired anterolisthesis, associated with degenerative changes, without an associated disruption or defect in the vertebral ring [1].

1.1.1. Etiopathogenesis

LDS affects predominantly the Caucasian population, mostly women above 50 years old. It is caused by severe degenerative disc and joint changes. The most frequent sliding is the anterolisthesis of the L4 on L5 (segment where the lumbar spine reaches the maximum level of lordosis), followed by the sliding of L3 on L4 and L5 on S1 [2].

Anatomical risk factors provoking LDS pathology can be: disc degeneration (this causes instability especially on the sagittal plane); sagittal orientation of the articular facets of the posterior apophysis; joint facet arthritis with loss of stability; increase in the angle between the peduncles and the facet joints; hypermobility due to muscle-ligament malfunction [3, 4, 5].

Lumbar degeneration can be described by the Kirkaldy-Willis degenerative process which occurs in progressive stages. During early stages, biochemical changes induce microscopic damage of the intervertebral disc. Subsequently, the height of the intervertebral disc decreases and the mechanical stress on the articular facets increases with reactive synovitis and progressive instability between adjacent vertebral bodies [6].

1.1.2. Classification

The historical classification of Wiltse, which was later modified by Ogilvie, classified the disease into degenerative, isthmic, dysplastic, traumatic, post-surgical/iatrogenic, or pathological.

Meyerding's classification assess the degree of vertebral sliding: grade 1 (0-25%); grade 2 (25-50%); grade 3 (50-75%); grade 4 (75-100%). It is still used to define the severity of listhesis. Grade 1 represents roughly 75% of all cases and LDS rarely exceeds grade 2 [7].

More recent classifications introduce concepts related to the spino-pelvic balance and global sagittal balance.

Gille classifies LDS into 3 types by evaluating: SL (Segmental Lordosis), LL (Lumbar Lordosis), PI (Pelvic Incidence), PT (Pelvic Tilt), and SVA (Sagittal Vertical Axis) [8].

CARDS (Clinical And Radiological Degenerative Spondylolisthesis) classification system identifies 4 types of spondylolisthesis by evaluating the disc space, the vertebral translation, and sagittal alignment [9].

1.1.3. Clinical Scenarios

LDS can be completely asymptomatic going unnoticed throughout life or conversely emerge following the development of other lumbar pathologies, such as the onset of a symptomatic disc herniation, a lumbar canal stenosis, a degenerative scoliosis.

Symptomatology can be centred in the lumbar region, or it can be represented by the association of LBP (Low Back Pain) and/or radicular deficit, up to, in case of stenosis, neurogenic claudication. Therefore, the term lumbo-sciatica indicates a lumbar pain that radiates to the limb or lower limbs with sciatic distribution L5 and/or S1; the term lumbo-cruralgia means a lumbo-sacral pain radiated in the territory of the femoral nerve (L3 - inguinal area, L4 - anterior face of the thigh).

LBP is a mechanical symptom linked to vertebral instability and is an indicator of chronicity. It is characterized by a severe pain during prolonged standing or physical exertion. Pain tends to disappear with rest and lying down.

As already mentioned above, LDS can cause central and/or lateral lumbar stenosis, affecting one or more roots of the cauda equina, which in turn can also be unilateral or bilateral. Stenosis is due to the sliding and/or the compression by disc bulging, by joint hypertrophy and ligamentous disfunction.

Central or mixed lumbar stenosis generally determines a neurological claudication or intermittent lumbar-radicular claudication: the patient at rest does not have radicular disorders; the patient, during prolonged walking, presents paraesthesia or asthenia to one or both lower limbs. In this latter case, the individual might experience a severe loss of walking autonomy (even below 50 meters). If the patient stops walking or sits down, the complaints disappear relatively quickly and reappear when resuming a prolonged walk.

It is differentiated from vascular claudication because the patient does not need to massage his/her legs.

Claudication is caused by the ischemic suffering of spinal roots, which in turn leads to a reduction of nerve impulses in the lower limbs.

Lateral stenosis in particular can cause unilateral or bilateral claudication, often characterized by limping. In most cases stenosis generates continuous radicular pain accentuated by walking.

With progression of the disease, neurological deficits such as loss of sensitivity, reflexes, and/or strength may also occur. Rarely, a cauda equina syndrome with sphincter deficiency (urinary/faecal incontinence), erectile dysfunction, and/or saddle paraesthesia (perineum and perianal region), is observed, usually following an acute herniated disc.

To summarize, radiculopathy is one of the most relevant clinical sign of LDS resulting from vertebral subluxation, disc degeneration and the consequent foraminal and/or central stenosis.

1.1.4. Clinical Examination and Imaging

The anamnesis and physical examination will allow the physician to obtain most of the necessary information to trace the possible cause of the LBP [10].

Low back pain has several causes and its prevalence is very high within the population. Chronic forms affect about 20% of the global population and a significant portion of this percentage is affected by LDS [11-12].

Conditions that guide us towards a LDS are: adulthood; absence of recent trauma; mechanical characteristics of pain; neurologic claudication, radiculopathy, or both; absence of fever, weight loss, or other possible signs of cancer.

It begins with a segmental examination of the spine, assessing the mobility of the spine in all directions and at each vertebral segment level. The anterior flexion, extension, lateral inclination and rotation are evaluated. Pain levels and amplitude of the movements are assessed.

Secondly, the patient is asked to walk in order to find out a possible neurogenic claudication. In this context, the patient is also asked to walk on the toes and to walk on the heels for evaluating a strength deficit due, respectively, to the involvement of S1 and L4-L5. Once inspected, the physician can start the palpation: the patient should be bare chested in a prone position on the bed. The lumbar spine is palpated starting from the spinous apophysis of L4 to evaluate the possible presence of pressure pain along the spine.

Neurological examination is performed by examining sensation, strength and tendon reflexes. Furthermore, Lasègue test (for L5-S1) and Wasserman test (for L3-L4) are performed to assess the presence of pain.

According to imaging, diagnosis is mainly based on X-ray studies executed in the 2 standard projections and in a standing position. Once the LDS and its related symptoms have been identified, a dynamic radiological study, maximum flexion/extension (pre-load/post-load), may be useful for a possible surgical treatment.

MRI can help us to assess soft tissues and to identify disc degeneration, the decay of posterior joints, and the compression of the thecal sac and nerve roots (see Figure 1). It provides an overall picture of the lumbosacral column, highlighting any degenerative-arthritic states that can be also found in other spinal levels [13].

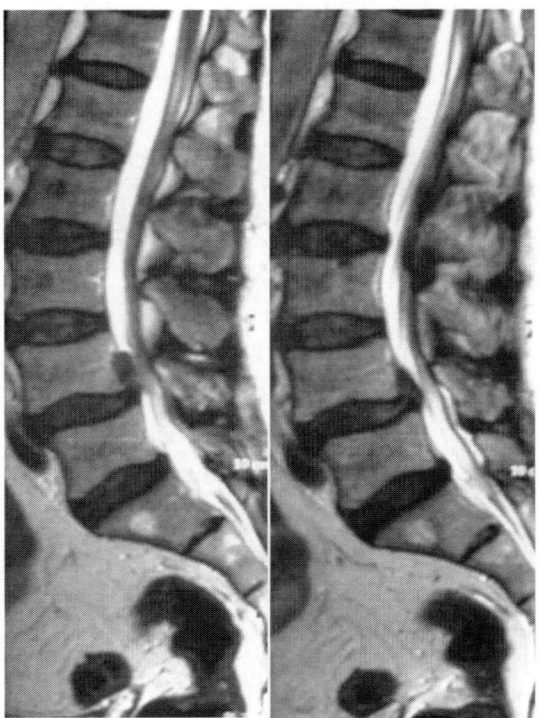

Figure 1. T2-weighted MRI images that show a Degenerative Spondylolisthesis of L4 on L5 with lumbar stenosis: in fact, in addition to a LBP, the patient had unilateral radiculopathy.

CT, on the other hand, can assess bone components and can demonstrate the presence of stenosis, vacuum discs, osteophytes, and loss of calcium tone. It is extremely useful for planning pedicle stabilization (pedicle and vertebral body length/width).

1.1.5. Functional Evaluation

Functional evaluation of a patient with LDS is based not only on the instrumental data but also various scales/scores, such as: VAS (Visual Analogue Scale) back and leg; ODI (Oswerty Disability Index); MacNab score.

VAS back and Leg are scales of evaluation of the subjective perception of pain intensity. It is a 10 cm line on which the patient records the level of pain experienced with a sign. The line is divided into 10 markers and labelled 0-10 (0 = no pain, 10 = worst possible pain).

ODI is a questionnaire that aims to assess the quality of life. It includes 10 elements which describe the level of disability (intensity of pain, personal care, lifting, walking, sitting, standing, sleeping, sex life, social life, and travelling). Each of the 10 elements includes a score from 0 to 5 to indicate its severity. The total score, which is the sum of all the points, is the Osweestry Disability Index.

A score between 0-20% indicates minimum disability, meaning that the patient can cope with most of life's activities. Usually no treatment is recommended and only postural advices are provided. A score between 21-40% indicates a moderate disability, so the patient feels more pain and has difficulty to sit, to stand up and to maintain an upright position. Pain can affect the patient's social and working life. Personal care, sexual activity and sleep are not seriously compromised and the patient can usually be managed conservatively. A score between 41-60% indicates a severe disability, thus pain remains the main problem and the activities of daily life are affected. These patients require detailed examination. A score between 61-80% indicates a disability: the back pain affects all aspects of the patient's life and a surgical treatment is usually required. A score between 81-100% indicates that the patient is bedridden.

MacNab criteria evaluates the patient' status after surgery. The outcome of the assessment can be: excellent (absence of pain, no limitation in movement, normal working activity possible); good (pain is present but not constant, possible to return to work, modest functional restrictions); fair (little functional improvement with some limitations on working and daily activities); poor (no improvement).

1.1.6. Treatment

LDS are usually asymptomatic or exhibit mild symptoms that do not require surgical treatment. Therefore, if there are no severe disorders (with or without neurological damage), the first therapeutic approach is conservative. Rehabilitation aims at strengthening the abdominal and paravertebral muscles by utilizing physical and postural exercises and anti-inflammatory drugs.

Even in the presence of a radiographic worsening, clinical symptoms can remain minor and only 30% of the cases would require surgery [14].

The surgical treatment must be only considered when severe/impair symptoms reduce the quality of life and do not respond to a conservative treatment of at least 3 months [15].

The purpose of surgery is to improve pain' symptomatology and any associated neurological deficits, in order to prevent further progression of deformity and to bring back a good sagittal and spino-pelvic balance (partially or totally reducing slipping). In the case of cauda equina syndrome, surgery becomes an urgent treatment [16].

The surgical options for patients with LDS are numerous. The operations are chosen accordingly to the surgeon's experience and his/her personal conduct and can be performed in an open or minimally invasive way.

The techniques for treating LDS can be: Posterior Decompression of the dural sac without arthrodesis (open or minimally invasive); Posterior Decompression with Posterolateral Fusion using bone graft; Posterior Decompression with instrumented Posterolateral Fusion; Posterior Stabilization without decompression (possibly percutaneously) with complete realignment (French School); Posterior Interbody Fusion (TLIF, PLIF) instrumented with or without decompression (possibly minimally invasive); Anterior/Anterolateral Interbody Fusion (ALIF, OLIF, XLIF) and indirect decompression with posterior time (with the only stabilization, possibly percutaneously); Anterior/Anterolateral Interbody Fusion (ALIF, OLIF, XLIF) and indirect decompression with posterior time (decompression and instrumented arthrodesis).

1.2. Minimally Invasive Transforaminal Approach

Traditionally, structural causes of LBP have been treated successfully with spinal fusion, which can be accomplished with a PLF (Postero-Lateral Fusion), PLIF (Posterior Lumbar Interbody Fusion), LLIF (Lateral Lumbar Interbody Fusion), ALIF (Anterior Lumbar Interbody Fusion) or OLIF (Oblique Lumbar Interbody Fusion).

The TLIF (Transforaminal Lumbar Interbody Fusion) approach was pioneered by Harms and Rolinger in 1982, with great success. The TLIF technique permits decompression of both central and foraminal stenosis as well as 3-column arthrodesis through a single posterior approach [17].

The traditional open TLIF (o-TLIF) requires a long, midline incision with dissection of the posterior tension band and bilateral paraspinal soft tissue for surgical exposure.

MI-TLIF is based on an interbody arthrodesis combined with the implantation of a posterior vertebral stabilization system which is inserted percutaneously.

Intervention steps will be the following: positioning; incision and localization; ipsilateral percutaneous placement of pedicle screws and rods; bony decompression; exposure of the thecal sac and disc space; discectomy, correction and interbody fusion.

The patient is intubated under general anesthesia and is placed prone onto a radiolucent operating table. Somatosensory Evoked Potentials (SSEPs) and Continuous Electromyographic Potentials (cEMG) are continuously monitored throughout the surgery. Triggered Electromyographic Potentials (tEMG) can be used to optionally test the needle, tap, and screw during pedicle cannulation. Under AP (anterior-posterior) fluoroscopic guidance, the midline over the spinous processes is outlined with a skin marker and 2 paramedian lines are drawn approximately 1 to 2 cm lateral to the lateral borders of the pedicles. The skin incisions are preliminarily swabbed with betadine. At this point, spinal needles are passed through the incisions bilaterally down to the pedicle entry points at the junction of the transverse process and the pedicle under AP fluoroscopy. Local anesthetics are used to inject the cylinder of soft tissue from these entry points, through the muscles and the skin itself, to reduce bleeding and postoperative pain. The patient is then prepped and draped in standard sterile fashion.

With lateral fluoroscopy, the initial tubular dilator is used to further localize and confirm the surgical level.

Skin incision, approximately 1.5 cm for peduncle, is performed along the intra-peduncular line with a scalpel about 3 cm long through the dermis, subcutaneous tissue, and fascia. Blunt dissection with fingers can be used to split the plane further and to bilaterally palpate the transverse process-facet junctions of the superior and inferior levels.

The opening of the fascia and separation of the paraspinal muscles is obtained through special dilators. Under fluoroscopic guidance, two Jamshidi needles (cannulated trocars) are inserted through the incisions, again down to the level of the pedicle entry points of the superior vertebral level at approximately the 3 o'clock and 9 o'clock positions of the pedicle. Needle follows the pedicle path beyond the posterior wall of the vertebral body. Each needle is then advanced approximately 2 cm through the incisions, taking care to not pass beyond the medial border of the circular pedicle projection on AP fluoroscopy to the corresponding 9 o'clock and 3 o'clock positions. Pedicle entry points should be placed more lateral and inferior along the pedicle such as to ensure that the screw head stays well away from the facet complex, to avoid adjacent facet impingement. At this depth in most patients, the needles typically end in the posterior third of the vertebral bodies on lateral fluoroscopy. At this point, vertebral body bone marrow aspiration can be performed after pedicle cannulation, with the osteoprogenitor cellular concentrate then admixed into an appropriate matrix to be combined with bone to be saved from the decompression.

The cannulated Jamshidi needles are removed after inserting the K-wires that will direct the final pedicle screw. A tap is placed over the K-wire to create a working channel, followed by placement of the percutaneous screw (see Figure 2). The process of tapping should be monitored with fluoroscopic guidance. Triggered Electromyographic Potentials stimulation of the tap and/or screw can be used at this point with plastic insulation sleeves to ensure that impedance is higher than 11 to 12 mA.

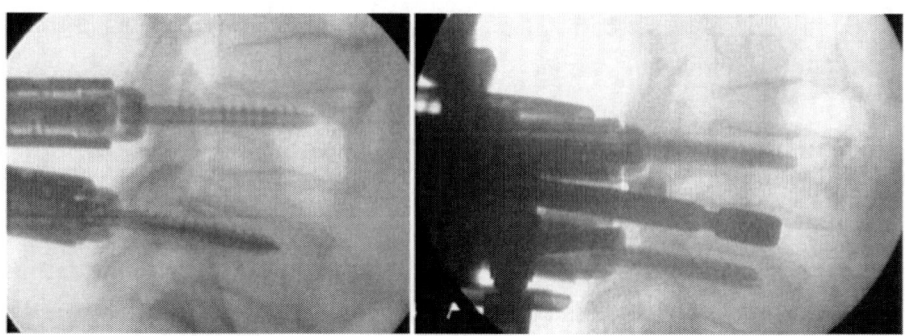

Figure 2. MI-TLIF approach. Operative control of the insertion of the pedicle screws with their percutaneous cannulas.

Tactile feedback plays an important role in the percutaneous cannulation of the peduncles; spongy osseous tissue of the peduncle is relatively soft and should allow regular needle advancement without obstacles related to the hardness of the cortical bone of the lateral and medial walls of the peduncle itself. Medial or lateral mispositioning of a pedicle screw is possible and may results in post-operative pain. It carries a need for immediate surgical revision.

Initially, minimally invasive pedicle screws with sleeve extenders are placed only contralateral to the side of the planned lamino-facetectomy decompression (ie, left-sided screws for a right-sided TLIF).

The same sequence of targeting, cannulation, K-wire placement, stimulation, tapping, and screw placement is then repeated for the inferior level.

Using the original contralateral incision, an appropriately sized rod is placed with a 90° handle, and passed underneath the fascia and through the polyaxial pedicle screw heads. Set screws are then placed through the pedicle screw extenders to secure the rod in place. For cases of mobile spondylolisthesis, the reduction mechanisms of several commercially available Minimally Invasive Spinal (MIS) screw systems will often be used at this point to partially or completely reduce the listhesis.

In cases where there is a more rigid slip and/or the presence of osteoporosis, aggressive reduction should be avoided at this point pending additional release of the facet joints during decompression. The ipsilateral K-wires are then angled away from the incisions and stapled to the surgical drape to provide access for the decompression portal.

A K-wire is placed onto the ipsilateral facet joint. Lateral fluoroscopy is used to confirm the correct surgical level and angle for surgical approach to the disc space. Sequential muscle-splitting tubular dilators are placed until the final static tubular or expandable retractor is locked into place with the flexible retractor arm between the K-wires. Bipolar cautery is first used to circumferentially coagulate the soft tissue vasculature around the edges of the tubular retractor. Monopolar electrocautery is then used to remove the soft tissue overlying the facet joint and the lamina. An up-angled curette is used to define the sublaminar plane. The lateral border of the facet, with particular focus on the pars interarticularis, is identified. A hemilaminotomy is performed with Kerrison rongeurs up to the rostral pedicle and down to the caudal pedicle. The remainder of the facet joint may be resected with rongeurs, osteotomes, or a pneumatic drill bit. Hemostasis is achieved with bone wax and thrombin-soaked gelfoam.

The ligamentum flavum is carefully resected to expose the underlying thecal sac. The thecal sac is decompressed from the central canal laterally until the traversing nerve root is clearly identified. Facet joint and ligament resection should be performed as far lateral as possible to provide an optimal angle of approach for the discectomy and interbody fusion. Autograft from the bony decompression is saved for fusion material, and can be combined with osteoconductive material and vertebral body bone marrow aspiration obtained earlier during pedicle cannulation. Typically, local bone graft, extender matrix and concentrated aspirate can be combined to obtain around 15 to 20 mL of composite graft material. In cases where there is severe bilateral central recess and foraminal stenosis, the working portal is angled such that decompression can be carried underneath the spinous process to achieve a contralateral laminectomy, facetectomy, and foraminotomy.

The disc is incised with a long-handled scalpel, and the discectomy is performed with a combination of curettes and pituitary rongeurs. If necessary, a nerve-root retractor is placed medially to gently retract the traversing nerve root and thecal sac to expose the underlying disc. Meticulous removal of the cartilaginous endplates will ensure the largest surface area available for bony fusion. With meticulous use of angled instruments, approximately 60% to 80% of the disc space can be effectively prepared for arthrodesis through a unilateral approach.

Sequentially larger disc space shavers are used to assist with the discectomy and preparation of the endplates for fusion. Blunt interbody dilators can also be used to progressively distract severely collapsed disc spaces, to restore the intervertebral height and facilitate the insertion of interbody discectomy tools. Particular attention should be paid to avoid using blunt dilators to distract the soft central area of the vertebral endplate, where inadvertent bony cavitation can occur. The dilator should be advanced cautiously such that distraction occurs primarily along the central far anterior ring hypophysis, where the endplate strength is maximal. During interbody paddle distraction, the contralateral screws can also be simultaneously distracted and the rod temporarily locked to maintain the increased interbody height to facilitate optimal cage height placement. Furthermore, several MIS pedicle screw systems have reduction threads or mechanisms to also reduce the spondylolisthesis at this moment, as the distraction typically mobilizes and releases the segment. This combined maneuver of ipsilateral interbody paddle height elevation, and contralateral screw distraction with reduction as needed, has been highly effective at correcting the slip and lordosis in most grade 2 and lower spondylolisthesis cases treated by the authors. The interbody cage and the disc space are then packed with the previously mentioned composite bone graft. Bone morphogenetic protein (BMP) may also be used with caution to ensure that the bioactive material remains anterior in the disc space, and that the annulotomy is well sealed at the end with fibrin glue and gelfoam to avoid unwanted leakage with subsequent radiculitis, seromas, and possible delayed heterotopic bone formation.

The cage is placed into the prepared disc space under fluoroscopic guidance to ensure that the graft is near the center as well as resting fully on the anterior ring hypophysis, to minimize the risk of delayed subsidence through the softer, center portion of the vertebral endplates. Hemostasis is achieved with an absorbable gelatin sponge and bipolar cautery of the epidural veins and soft tissue followed by antibiotic irrigation. A piece of gelfoam is placed within the annulotomy and sealed with fibrin glue if desired to prevent leakage of bone marrow and bioactive materials from the interbody space. The ipsilateral working portal is then carefully removed to avoid inadvertent removal of the ipsilateral K-wires within the pedicles.

The previously stapled ipsilateral K-wires are then released, and the pedicle screws with their extender sleeves are placed over them and threaded into the vertebral bodies. An ipsilateral rod is then introduced as was performed with the contralateral screws previously. When both rods are secured, bilateral compression is applied to the construct, before final locking of the set screws to maximize segmental lordosis and improve overall sagittal balance. Radiographs are used to confirm appropriate final placement of bilateral screws and rods (see Figure 3). Either a small handheld retractor or tubular portal is then placed down through the contralateral incision between the MIS pedicle extension sleeves. In this fashion, the contralateral facet and transverse processes can be decorticated and irrigated, with the remaining bone graft used to pack the bony posterolateral gutter. The MIS pedicle screw extension sleeves and the contralateral retractor are then all removed, leaving the final construct in place. The wounds are irrigated and closed with a combination of absorbable sutures and a skin adhesive for an optimal cosmetic closure. At this point, reinjection of local anesthetic into the skin and underlying muscle will help decrease postoperative pain [18-19-20].

To conclude, with this technique we obtain a 360° stabilization of the spine.

The aim of the study is to evaluate the clinical and functional results in the short and long term of MI-TLIF approach in the surgical treatment of LDS.

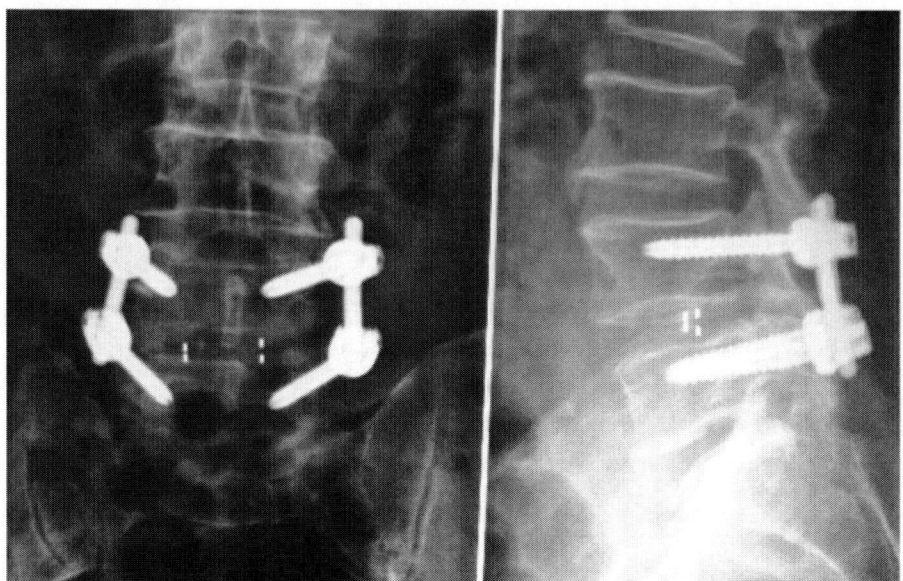

Figure 3. MI-TLIF approach. Final radiograms showing the correct positioning of the posterior vertebral stabilization system, consisting of screws and rods, and the interbody fusion cage (called also TLIF).

2. METHODS

A prospective observational study was conducted on a cohort of 23 patients, operated between 2014 and 2018, with MI-TLIF technique at the Orthopaedics and Traumatology department of the Policlinico Umberto I of Rome and ICOT of Latina.

In each patient the level of anterolisthesis and the presence of a lumbar stenosis and/or herniated disc were verified. Operative data (operative time, estimated blood loss), length of hospitalization and complications were assessed. In the pre-operative and in the FUP (follow-up), VAS (Visual Analogue Scale) and ODI (Oswestry Disability Index) were calculated. During the FUP, Radiographic check, MacNab score and Patient Satisfaction were also evaluated.

Initially, patients without worsening neurological deficits underwent 3 months of FKT (physiokinesitherapy).

Surgery was carried out in patients with: 3 months of FKT without improvement; a VAS back ≥ 6; a VAS leg ≥ 6; an ODI ≥ 50%.

The aim of this study is to evaluate the clinical and functional results in the short and long term of MI-TLIF. For this purpose the VAS back, VAS leg, and the ODI were evaluated in the pre-operative and in the post-operative (at 3 months, 1 year, and subsequently every year).

The inclusion criteria included indication for surgery and involvement of a single segment. The exclusion criteria included cancer and ongoing pregnancy.

3. RESULTS

Statistical analysis was carried out using the SPSS software (Statistical Package for Social Science). Continuous variables were reported as a mean with SD (standard deviation). Evaluation of the differences between continuous variables with normal distribution was assessed using a t-test for paired data. A p value < 0.05 was considered to be statistically significant.

Table 1. Characteristics of recruited patients

Variable	Patients undergoing MI-TLIF surgery (n=23)
Age (means ± SD), years	47 ± 8.7
Male/Female, n (%)	18/5 (78.3/21.7)
Symptomatology LBP, Low Back Pain Neurogenic claudication, stenosis Unilateral radiculopathy, hernia	n (%) 10 (43.5) 8 (34.8) 5 (21.7)
LDS level L3 - L4 L4 - L5 L5 - S1	n (%) 2 (8.7) 18 (78.3) 3 (13)
Pre-operative VAS back (mean ± SD)	7.3 ± 0.6
Pre-operative VAS leg (mean ± SD)	7.7 ± 0.8
Pre-operative ODI (mean ± SD), %	67 ± 10.8

The 23 patients had a mean age of 47 ± 8.7 years, of which 15 were males and 8 were female. They underwent clinical functional evaluation using VAS back, VAS leg, and ODI.

The evaluation was performed in the pre-operative and on FUP at 3 months, 1 year and 2 years following the intervention.

In the pre-operative the VAS back had a mean of 7.3 ± 0.6, the VAS leg had a mean of 7.7 ± 0.8 and the ODI had a mean of 67% ± 10.8%

The 23 patients (see Table 1) underwent MI-TLIF surgery combined with the implant of a posterior vertebral stabilization system.

Ten patients (43.5%) had only LBP, eight patients (34.8%) showed neurogenic claudication (stenosis), five patients (21.7%) had a unilateral radiculopathy (hernia).

Operation was performed on a single level: 18 (78.3%) at the L4-L5 level, 3 (13.0%) at the L5-S1 level and 2 (8.7%) at the L3-L4 level.

Mean operative time was 170 ± 22.3 minutes, while the mean blood loss was 205 ± 38.2 ml.

Mean of hospitalization time was 5 ± 1.6 days. No patient needed transfusion and none had infections. Three patients (13%), operated on L4-L5, showed a unilateral sensory/motor radicular deficit from the insertion side of the TLIF cage. However, this acquired neurological deficit was temporary, in fact, after 6 months, the 3 patients no longer had radiculopathy.

Three months after surgery, the mean of VAS back was 2.7 ± 0.7, the mean of VAS leg was 4.7 ± 1.9, and the mean of ODI was 37 ± 17.5%.

One year after the surgery, the mean of VAS back was 2.75 ± 0.4, the mean of VAS leg was 3.0 ± 0.6, and the mean of ODI was 32 ± 9.3%.

Two years after the surgery, the mean of VAS back was 2.8 ± 0.7, the mean of VAS leg was 3.8 ± 1.1, and the mean of ODI was 35 ± 10.7%.

The difference seen between the means of the VAS back variable in the 4 times was assessed through the t-test. A statistically significant difference emerged from this comparison (p = 0.045) (see Table 2, Figure 4).

The difference between the means of the variable VAS leg in the 4 times was compared by t-test. This was also statistically significant (p = 0.018) (see Table 2, Figure 4).

The difference between the means of the ODI variables was analysed through the t-test. Also from this comparison, a statistically significant difference (p = 0.013) (see Table 2, Figure 4).

Furthermore, at 3 months, 1 year and subsequently, the Radiographic check did not show implantation problems. In the FUP, MacNab criteria was also evaluated: 78.3% of the patients obtained a good outcome and 21.7% a fair outcome. Patient Satisfaction was 78.3% of 23 patients (18 patients were satisfied with the treatment received and they would undergo surgery again).

Table 2. Representation of the VAS back, VAS leg and ODI values in the 4 times. Data are reported as mean ± standard deviation (SD). The level of statistical significance (p) was obtained through t-test for paired data

Variable	mean ± SD	p
vas back		
pre-operative	7.3 ± 0.6	
3 months	2.7 ± 0.7	0.045
1 year	2.5 ± 0.4	
2 years	2.8 ± 0.7	
vas leg		
pre-operative	7.7 ± 0.8	
3 months	4.7 ± 1.9	0.018
1 year	3 ± 0.6	
2 years	3.8 ± 1.1	
odi (%)		
pre-operative	67 ± 10.8	
3 months	37 ± 17.5	0.013
1 year	32 ± 9.3	
2 years	35 ± 10.7	

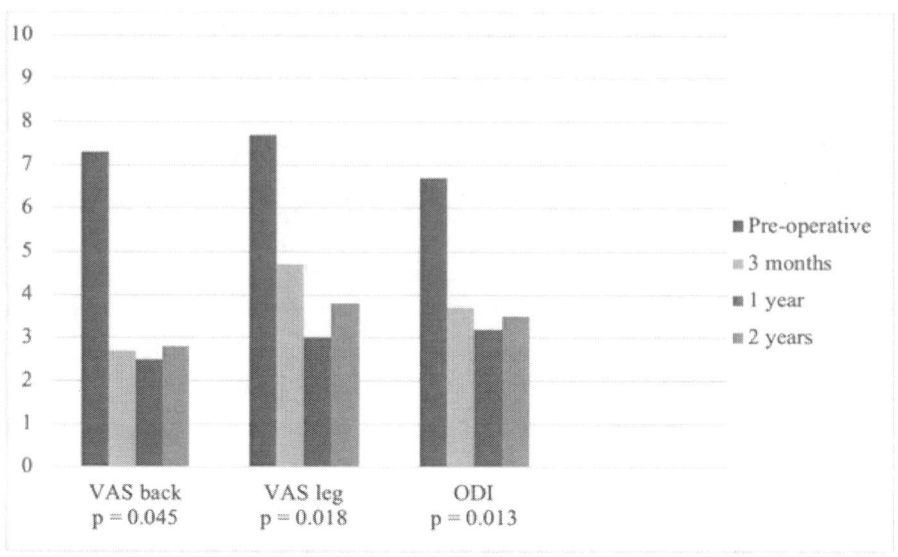

Figure 4. Histogram representing the distribution of the mean of the VAS back, VAS leg and ODI values in the 4 times. The level of statistical significance (p) was obtained through t-test for paired data.

4. DISCUSSION

MISS (Minimally Invasive Spine Surgery) allows you to treat many pathological conditions of the spine with day surgery or very short hospitalizations. With MISS it is possible to perform the same surgical gestures performed in open procedures obtaining decompressions and stabilizations of the spine.

Percutaneous techniques (p-MISS) are included in the field of minimally invasive interventions, which denote: better cosmetics, as the surgical incision is limited to a few millimetres; less impact on fascial, tendinous and muscle structures; limited blood loss; reduced risk of infection; shorter hospitalization times; reduced use of analgesic drugs; rapid functional recovery [18, 19, 20].

According to the literature, the data of this analysis shows that MI-TLIF, with the posterior vertebral stabilization system, can optimize hospitalization times and functional recovery, thanks to the reduced surgical invasiveness and the lower impact on surrounding structures.

In the post-operative, the most frequent complication was radicular pain on the side of the cage insertion, due to the manipulation and spreading of the spinal roots. In fact, the operating space is narrow and the placement of the cage is complex. The neurological deficit occurs especially in L4-L5 or more cranially.

The aim of the study is to use VAS back, VAS leg and ODI to compare the quality of life of patients before and after MISS. In addition, operative data, length of hospitalization and any complications were evaluated. MacNab criteria and Patient Satisfaction were also recorded in the FUP to analyse and understand the level of patient' status.

From the analysis of the VAS back and leg scales as well as the ODI, statistically significant differences emerged in the comparison of the means in the pre-operative and FUP results. Especially, more than satisfactory results have emerged in the FUP at 3 months, results that suggest that the mini-invasiveness of this intervention can be related to excellent results in the short term.

Overall, MI-TLIF approach showed satisfying clinical results, an optimization of hospitalization times and functional recovery, as well as limited bleeding and a reduced infection rate, thanks to the reduced surgical invasiveness and the reduced damage induced on the paravertebral muscles and soft tissues. In addition, despite the possible post-operative root suffering, the technique can be considered safe and effective as proved in more than 80% of our patients.

REFERENCES

[1] Matz P, Meagher RJ, Lamer T, et al. Diagnosis and Treatment of Degenerative Lumbar Spondylolisthesis (2014) *Evidence-Based Clinical Guidelines for Multidisciplinary Spine Care.* North American Spine Society.

[2] Wang YXJ, Káplár Z, Deng M, et al. (2017) Lumbar degenerative spondylolisthesis epidemiology: A systematic review with a focus on gender-specific and age-specific prevalence. *Journal of Orthopaedic Translation* 11:39-52.

[3] Sengupta DK, Herkowitz HN. (2005) Degenerative Spondylolisthesis: Review of Current Trends and Controversies. *Spine* 30(Suppl):S71-81.

[4] DeVine JG, Schenk-Kisser JM, Skelly AC. (2012) Risk factors for degenerative spondylolisthesis: a systematic review. *Evid Based Spine Care J.;* 3(2):25-34.

[5] Cinotti G, Postacchini F, Fassari F, et al. (1997) Predisposing factors in degenerative spondylolisthesis. A radiographic and CT study. *Int Orthop.;* 21(5):337-342.

[6] Slikker W.III, Espinoza Orías AA, Shifflett GD, et al. (2020) Image-Based Markers Predict Dynamic Instability in Lumbar Degenerative Spondylolisthesis. *Neurospine* 17(1)221-227.

[7] Alfieri A, Gazzeri R, Prell J et al. (2013) The current management of lumbar spondylolisthesis. *J Neurosurg Sci.;* 57(2):103-113.

[8] Gille O, Bouloussa H, Mazas S et al. (2017) A new classification system for degenerative spondylolisthesis of the lumbar spine. *Eur Spine J* 26:3096-3105.

[9] Sobol GL, Hilibrand A, Davis A, et al. (2018) Reliability and Clinical Utility of the CARDS Classification for Degenerative Spondylolisthesis. *Clin Spine Surg.* 31:E69-73.

[10] Matz PG, Meagher RJ, Lamer T, et al. (2016) Guideline summary review: An evidence-based clinical guideline for the diagnosis and treatment of degenerative lumbar spondylolisthesis. *Spine J.* 16(3):439-448.

[11] Bitenc-Jasiejko A, Konior K, Lietz-Kijak D. (2020) Meta-Analysis of Integrated Therapeutic Methods in Noninvasive Lower Back Pain Therapy (LBP): The Role of Interdisciplinary Functional Diagnostics. *Pain Research and Management.* 1-17.

[12] Kalichman L, Kim DH, Li L, et al. (2009) Spondylolysis and Spondylolisthesis: Prevalence and Association with Low Back Pain in the Adult Community-Based Population. *Spine* 34:199.

[13] Epstein NE, Hollingsworth RD. (2017) Nursing review of diagnosis and treatment of lumbar degenerative spondylolisthesis. *Surgical Neurology International.* 8:246.

[14] Kim K, Youn Y, Lee SH, et al. (2018) The Effectiveness and Safety of Nonsurgical Integrative Interventions for Symptomatic Lumbar Spinal Spondylolisthesis: A Randomized Controlled Multinational, Multicenter Trial Protocol. *Medicine* 97(19):e0667.

[15] Watters WC 3rd, Bono CM, Gilbert TJ, et al. (2009) An evidence-based clinical guideline for the diagnosis and treatment of degenerative lumbar spondylolisthesis. *Spine J.* 9(7):609-614.

[16] Eismont FJ, Norton RP, Hirsch BP. (2014) Surgical Management of Lumbar Degenerative Spondylolisthesis. *Journal of the American Academy of Orthopaedic Surgeons* 22(4):203-213.

[17] Harms J, Rolinger H. (1982) A one-stage procedure in operative treatment of spondylolistheses: dorsal traction-reposition and anterior fusion (author's transl). *Z Orthop Ihre Grenzgeb* 120:343-347.

[18] Wong AP, Smith ZA, Stadler JA et al. (2014)Minimally Invasive Transforaminal Lumbar Interbody Fusion (MI-TLIF): Surgical Technique, Long-Term 4-year Prospective Outcomes, and Complications Compared With an Open TLIF Cohort. *Neurosurg Clin N Am.* 25(2):279-304.

[19] Mobbs RJ, Sivabalan P, Li J. (2011) Technique, challenges and indications for percutaneous pedicle screw fixation. *Journal of Clinical Neuroscience.* 18:741-749.

[20] Harris EB, Massey P, Lawrence J, et al. (2008) Percutaneous techniques for minimally invasive posterior lumbar fusion. *Neurosurg Focus.* 25(2):E12.

BIOGRAPHICAL SKETCH

Alessandro Ramieri

Affiliation: Faculty of Pharmacy and Medicine, Department Orthopaedics and Traumatology. University "La Sapienza" of Rome, Italy

Education: Rome University "La Sapienza," Eurospine, AO Spine

Research and Professional Experience:

July 1995 – Graduate Medicine and Surgery Sapienza Rome University
July 1996-July 1997 – Medical Officer Italian Army
Nov 2002-present – Post-graduate Degree in Orthopaedics and Traumatology
Sapienza Rome University
May 2011 – PhD Pathophysiology and Muscle-Skeletal Disorders
Sapienza Rome University
May 2014-present – Research Fellow and Teacher,
Sapienza Rome University
Nov 2011 – European Spine Course Diploma (Budapest session)
Feb 2014 – Eurospine TFR Course Diploma (Dublin)
May 2000 – GIS-Italian Spine Society Member (Ordinary)
Apr 2014-present – AOSPINE Member (Silver)
Apr 2003- Mar 2004 – spinal surgeon S. Pertini Rome Hospital
Gen 2005-Apr 2018 – orthopaedic consultant Sapienza Polo Pontino ICOT, Latina
Gen 2005-present – orthopaedic consultant Don Gnocchi Onlus Foundation, Milan
Gen 2011-present – orthopaedic consultant Capodarco Onlus Foundation, Rome
Apr 2020-present – Resercher and Professor, University La Sapienza, Rome Italy

Scholastic screening for AIS prevention in 2002; Several projects in the field of spinal diseases for the Italian Ministry of Health from 2010 to 2015; Teacher and tutor in Master Courses on Mininvasive Techniques in Spinal Pathologies, S. Andrea Hosp, Sapienza University, Rome Italy; Tutor in the AOSpine course "Thoracolumbar Spine Stabilization," Rome 2014;

Teacher in "Neurophysiopathological Techniques," MIPAD Lazio, Sapienza Rome University, 2007-08

Editorial Board Member for WJO-World Journal of Orthopaedics; Editorial Board Member for JSM-Neurosurgery and Spine; Reviewer forWorld Journal Of Orthopedics, J. Neuroscience in Rural Practice, Neurosurgical Review, J Neurology Neurosugery and Psychiatry, Annals of case report, Annals of Orthopaedics, Journal of Pain Research, Scientific Journal of Neurology and Neurosurgery; Orth. Researc and Review (Dove Press)

Professional Appointments: AO International Validation Group on "AO Spine Subaxial Fractures classification system international validation study" e "AO Spine Sacral classification system validation study"

Honors:

1995 Tagliapietra Award, Sinch-Italian Neurosurgery Society; 2000 GIS Scholarship, GIS Italian Spine Society

Last 3 Years Publications:

1) Alessandro Ramieri, Giorgio Ippolito, Umberto Prencipe, Giovanni Corsini, Maurizio Domenicucci, Giuseppe Costanzo (2020): Chapter 34. Osteolytic Metastases of the Thoracolumbar Spine: The Role of the Vertebroplasty and Kyphoplasty. In: Landi A, Gregori F, Delfini R: *Spinal cord and spinal column tumors.* Nova Science Publishers, Inc., Hauppauge NY, 11788 USA, ISBN: 978-1-53616-474-9.
2) Miscusi M, Ramieri A, Forcato S, Trungu S, Domenicucci M, Costanzo G, Raco A (2020): Chapter 33: Minimally Invasive Spinal Surgery

(MISS) for Neurological Metastases of the Thoracic and Lumbar Spine. In: Landi A, Gregori F, Delfini R: *Spinal cord and spinal column tumors*. Nova Science Publishers, Inc., Hauppauge NY, 11788 USA, ISBN: 978-1-53616-474-9.

3) Ramieri A, Domenicucci M, Corsini G, Campopiano G, Miscusi M (2017). Anatomia funzionale e biomeccanica della giunzione cranio-spinale e del rachide cervicale sub-assiale. In: Delfini R, Landi A. (a cura di): Delfini R, Landi A, *La Chirurgia del Rachide Cervicale*. ROMA CIC Edizioni Internazionali, ISBN: 8893890054. [Functional and biomechanical anatomy of the cranio-spinal junction and sub-axial cervical spine. In: Delfini R, Landi A. (edited by): Delfini R, Landi A, *Cervical Spine Surgery*.]

4) Ramieri A, Polli FM, Manauzzi E, Meloncelli S, Costanzo G (2017). Fissaggio posteriore cervicale interfaccettale: il sistema DTRAX®. In: Delfini R, Landi A. (a cura di): Delfini R, Landi A, *La Chirurgia del Rachide Cervicale*. ROMA CIC Edizioni Internazionali, ISBN: 8893890054. [Posterior cervical interfacetal fixation: the DTRAX® system. In: Delfini R, Landi A. (edited by): Delfini R, Landi A, *Cervical Spine Surgery*.]

5) Spinal epidural hematomas: personal experience and literature review of more than 1000 cases M Domenicucci, C Mancarella, G Santoro, DE Dugoni, A Ramieri, ... *Journal of Neurosurgery: Spine* 27 (2), 198-208, 2017.

6) Comparison of pure lateral and oblique lateral inter-body fusion for treatment of lumbar degenerative disk disease: a multicentric cohort study M Miscusi, A Ramieri, S Forcato, M Giuffrè, S Trungu, M Cimatti, A Pesce, ... *European Spine Journal* 27 (2), 222-228, 2018.

7) Long-term clinical outcomes and quality of life in elderly patients treated with interspinous devices for lumbar spinal stenosis. M Miscusi, S Trungu, S Forcato, A Ramieri, FM Polli, A Raco. *Journal of Neurological Surgery Part A: Central European Neurosurgery* 79 (02 …, 2018.

8) Surgical management of coronal and sagittal imbalance of the spine without PSO: a multicentric cohort study on compensated adult

degenerative deformities. A Ramieri, M Miscusi, M Domenicucci, A Raco, G Costanzo. *European Spine Journal* 26 (4), 442-449, 2017.

9) Lumbar ganglion cyst: Nosology, surgical management and proposal of a new classification based on 34 personal cases and literature review. M Domenicucci, A Ramieri, D Marruzzo, P Missori, M Miscusi, R Tarantino, *World Journal of Orthopedics* 8 (9), 697, 2017.

10) Thoraco-lumbar fractures with blunt traumatic aortic injury in adult patients: correlations and management. G Santoro, A Ramieri, V Chiarella, M Vigliotta, M Domenicucci. *European Spine Journal* 27 (2), 248-257, 2018.

11) Miscusi M., Serrao M., Conte C., Ippolito G., Marinozzi F., Bini F., Troise S., Forcato S., Trungu S., Ramieri A., Pierelli F., Raco A. (2019). Spatial and temporal characteristics of the spine muscles activation during walking in patients with lumbar instability due to degenerative lumbar disk disease: Evaluation in pre-surgical setting. *Human Movement Science,* vol. 66, p. 371-382, ISSN: 0167-9457, doi: 10.1016/j.humov.2019.05.013.

12) V Chiarella, A Ramieri, M Giugliano, M Domenicucci Rapid spontaneous resolution of lumbar ganglion cysts: A case report. *World Journal of Orthopedics* 11 (1): 68-75, 2020.

13) Massimo Miscusi, Alessandro Ramieri, Stefano Forcato, Sokol Trungu, Alessandro Pesce, Pietro Familiari, Giuseppe Costanzo, Antonino Raco (2019): Global Spine Congress, Toronto: Comparison of Clinical Outome and Spinopelvic Parameters Modifications Between Minimally Invasive and Conventional Open Posterior Lumbar Interbody Fusion for Treatment of High- Grade L5-S1 Isthmic Spondylolisthesis. *Global Spine Journal,* Vol. 9(2S) 2S-187S [a] The Author(s) 2019 Article reuse guidelines: sagepub.com/journals-permissions doi: 10.1177/219256821 9839730 journals.sagepub.com/home/gsj.

14) Alessandro Ramieri, Stefano Forcato, Sokol Trungu, Alessandro Pesce, Pietro Familiari, Massimo Miscusi, Giuseppe Costanzo, Antonino Raco (2019): Global Spine Congress, Toronto: Lateral Lumbar Inter-Body Fusion in Lumbar Adult Deformities: Fusion Rate and Results. *Global Spine Journal,* Vol. 9(2S) 2S-187S [a] The Author(s) 2019 Article reuse

guidelines: sagepub.com/journals-permissions doi: 10.1177/21925682 19839730 journals.sagepub.com/home/gsj.

15) Maurizio Domenicucci, Alessandro Ramieri (2018): Global Spine Congress, Singapore: Lumbar Ganglion Cyst: Nosology, Surgical Management And Proposal of a New Classification Based on 34 Personal Cases and Literature Review. *Global Spine Journal,* Vol. 8(1S) 2S-173S [a] The Author(s) 2018 Reprints and permission: sagepub.com/journals Permissions.nav doi: 10.1177/21925682187710 30 journals.sagepub.com/home/gsj.

16) Alessandro Ramieri, Giuseppe Costanzo, Massimo Miscusi, Antonino Raco (2018): Restoring Lumbar Lordosis and Balance of the Spine without Pso or Vcr: Multicentric Experience on a Cohort of 50 Consecutive Adult Degenerative Kyphoscoliosis. *Global Spine Journal,* Vol. 8(1S) 174S-374S [a] The Author(s) 2018 Reprints and permission: sagepub.com/journals Permissions.nav doi: 10.1177/2192568218771 072 journals.sagepub.com/home/gsj.

17) Alessandro Ramieri, Giuseppe Costanzo (2018): FMwand in Posterior and Lateral Surgery for Spinal Deformities: Clinical and Radiological Study. *Global Spine Journal,* Vol. 8(1S) 174S- 374S [a] The Author(s) 2018 Reprints and permission: sagepub.com/journals Permissions.nav doi: 10.1177/2192568218771072 journals.sagepub.com/home/gsj.

18) Giorgio Santoro, Alessandro Ramieri, Maurizio Domenicucci: Global Spine Congress, Singapore: Thoraco-Lumbar Fractures With Traumatic Aortic Injury (TAI) in Adult Patients: Classification and Management. *Global Spine Journal* 2018, Vol. 8(1S) 2S-173S [a] The Author(s) 2018 Reprints and permission: sagepub.com/journals Permissions.nav doi: 10.1177/2192568218771030.

19) Massimo Miscusi, Stefano Forcato, Filippo Maria Polli, Alessandro Ramieri, Marco Cimatti, Giuseppe Costanzo, Antonino Raco (2017): Global Spine Congress, Milano: Pure Lateral and Oblique Lateral Interbody Fusion for Treatment of Lumbar Degenerative Disk Disease: Comparison of Two Different Techniques. *Global Spine Journal,* Vol. 7(2S) 2S-189S [a] The Author(s) 2017 Reprints and permission:

sagepub.com/journals Permissions.nav doi: 10.1177/2192568217708577 journals.sagepub.com/home/gsj.

20) Alessandro Ramieri, Massimo Miscusi, Filippo Maria Polli, Giuseppe Costanzo (2017): Global Spine Congress, Milano: Safety and Efficacy of Multilevel XLIFs Approaching the Convex Side of Adult Scoliosis Above 30 Degrees. *Global Spine Journal*, Vol. 7(2S) 2S-189S [a] The Author(s) 2017 Reprints and permission: sagepub.com/journals Permissions.nav doi: 10.1177/2192568217708577 journals.sagepub.com/home/gsj.

21) Sokol Trongu, Massimo Miscusi, Luca Ricciardi, Stefano Forcato, Alessandro Ramieri, Antonino Raco. The ante-psoas approach (ATP) for interbody fusion at the L5-S1 segment: clinical and radiological outcomes [FOCUS20-335R1]. *J Neurosurgical Focus* (in press).

Chapter 4

Minimally Invasive vs Conventional Open Posterior Lumbar Interbody Fusion in the Treatment of High-Grade L5 Isthmic Spondylolisthesis

Alessandro Ramieri[1,*], *MD, PhD,*
Massimo Miscusi[2], *MD, PhD, Sokol Trungu*[2], *MD,*
Stefano Forcato[3], *MD, Amedeo Piazza*[2], *MD,*
Antonino Raco[2], *MD and Giuseppe Costanzo*[1], *MD*

[1]Rome Italy, Faculty of Pharmacy and Medicine,
Dpt Orthopaedics and Traumatology, University "La Sapienza"
[2]Rome Italy, NESMOS Sant'Andrea Hospital,
University "La Sapienza"
[3]Tricase, Lecce Italy Neurosurgery, G. Panico Hospital

---

[*] Corresponding Author's E-mail: alexramieri@libero.it

Abstract

Purpose: To compare the effectiveness and changes of the spino-pelvic parameters between the minimally invasive PLIF and traditional posterior open approach in the treatment of a prospective randomized series of high-grade adult isthmic spondylolisthesis (HGISL). Material and Methods: Two homogeneous groups of 14 adult patients with a painful high-grade isthmic L5 spondylolisthesis (Meyerding III or IV) were operated by open (group A) and minimally invasive PLIF (MISS group B). L4-S1 instrumentation and L5-S1 interbody fusion were realized. Deformities were classified according to the SDSG, measuring slippage, slip angle, thoracic kyphosis (TK), lumbar lordosis (LL), sagittal vertical axis (SVA), pelvic tilt (PT). A PT value $\leq 30°$ was assumed as a condition of balanced pelvis. Clinical evaluation was based on the back and leg VAS, ODI and SF36. Results: Mean age was 24 (range 19-39), with F:M ratio 2.5:1. Seven deformities were type 7 and 21 type 8. We had 7% of early major neurological complications, Blood loss was greater in group A (p 0.037), as the hospital length (p = 0.02). At follow-up (mean 29.4, range 24-42), radiographic and clinical parameters overall improved ($p < 0.05$), without significant differences between groups ($p > 0.05$). The PT decreased below 30° degrees in 9 type 8 HGISL. The SVA moved slightly forward and LL showed a little reduction ($p > 0.05$). A slip angle >10° was related to the worst clinical follow-up painful condition ($p < 0.03$). Conclusion: As in other spinal diseases, the posterior MISS seems to be non-inferior to open approach in the HGISL surgical care. MISS was better in relation to the estimated blood loss and hospital lenght. Changes of spino-pelvic parameters were observed in both procedures, but further studies will be required to demonstrate a clear correlation between radiological and clinical results. Data showed that our estimated parameters did not significantly affect the clinical outcomes as measured at the last follow-up, except for the slip angle.

Keywords: isthmic spondylolisthesis, adult spine deformity, posterior fusion, minimally invasive surgery

1. Introduction

In the dysplastic lumbo-sacral spondylolisthesis, the slip severity is usually classified using the Meyerding method [1]. High-grade slips are those with more than 50% slippage. In the general population, the prevalence of slip progression is low and has been found to decrease with increasing age [2-4]. Such a condition is cause of low-back pain and radicular signs due to narrowing of segmental neural foramina. In case of high-grade slippage, pelvic parameters can be severely affected leading to a severe sagittal deformity, with or without unbalance of the whole spine [5, 6]. Surgery is recommended when low-back pain episodes and/or radicular symptoms become frequent and refractory to medical and physical treatments. If the aims of surgery have been clearly defined, including the lythic inflammatory tissue removal, extensive opening of the neural foramen with root neurolysis and fusion, the real need to correct slipping is still extensively debated, especially in adults, whose "structured" deformity is harshly reduced, in comparison to those of the young individuals, because of different tissue elasticity and compliance [7].

1.1. Open Surgery and Minimally Invasive Surgery: Technical Notes

Open surgery consisted of a median supraspinous traditional approach, paravertebral muscle dissection and L5 posterior neural arch total resection. A complete neurolysis and visualization of L5 and S1 nerve roots were mandatory to decrease neurological risks during PLIF. After screw positioning, a dedicated retractor supported by the screw heads was used to spread the intervertebral space first on one side and then contralaterally. Bilateral radical diskectomy was achieved to allocate cages. When required, osteotomy of the sacral dome was performed to ameliorate the vertebral body mobility and reducibility. Final compression fixation was performed by lordotic rods finally locked with the patient's hips in extension position.

In the MISS procedure, percutaneous screws were inserted. A bilateral mini-open Wiltse approach, performed by a four-handed technique, realized 3 main advantages: a reduction of paravertebral muscles resistance and damage, an ideal angle for screws and cages insertion, a safer bilateral arthrectomy and foraminotomy using the intraoperative microscope, After the bilateral radical disk excision, a progressive mobilization of the vertebral endplates was done using shavers and Cobbs simultaneously in both sides. Sometimes, sacral dome osteotomy was used to increase reduction. One-side straight rod insertion allowed the partial reduction of the slippage and PLIF-shaped cage was inserted through opening of the disk from the opposite site. Once the first cage was placed, the straight rod was removed from one side and mounted on the opposite side to complete the segmental correction. A second PLIF-shaped cage was then inserted as well as the final lordotic rods. With the patient's hips extension, the final compression fixation was obtained to recover the most lordosis as possible.

2. METHODS

Based on the literature data, mainly concerning low-grade and only occasionally HGISL case reports or small cohorts [8-11], that seem to prove the effectiveness of the minimally invasive spine surgery (MISS), as much the traditional open surgery can do, we planned to investigate if MISS could also play a role in the treatment of high-grade isthmic spondylolisthesis (HGISL).

We realized an observational study by prospective data on a multicentric homogeneous case series obtained from the adult population with a HGISL, comparing clinical outcomes and modifications of the spinal and pelvic parameters achieved by open and MISS surgery. Furthermore, we hypothesized that the final clinical results were affected by an imperfect spino-pelvic balance.

Twenty-eight consecutive adult patients with symptomatic, unresponsive to minimum six-months of conservative treatments, high dysplastic L5 HGISL were prospectively enrolled in the period between January 2014 and November 2017. Final cohort were operated in three different hospitals. We used the Spinal Deformity Study Group (SDSG) classification [12] to typify the lumbo-sacral deformity. Cases with unbalance of the spine were excluded. Patients were …. divided in two groups according to the surgical procedure: 14 patients were operated by conventional open surgery (group A) and other 14 by MISS procedure (group B). Results were subsequently compared in terms of postoperative changes in spinal and spino-pelvic parameters and improvement of clinical outcomes. In order to minimize bias, all patients included underwent an L5-S1 interbody fusion using PLIF-shaped cages and L4-S1 posterior pedicle screw fixation. In this way, we obtained two homogeneous series for demographic, clinical, radiological and surgical characteristics.

Intraoperative and post-operative data, as well as complications, were collected. Clinical evaluations were performed applying back and leg VAS, ODI and Short Form 36 – Physical Component Summary (SF-36 PCS) at baseline, postoperatively (1 month/3 months) and after a minimum of 2 years follow-up. Spinal and spino-pelvic parameters were evaluated in both groups before and after surgery, by a comparison between preoperative and postoperative full-spine standing x-rays. The analyzed radiographic measures were: sagittal vertebral axis (SVA), lumbar lordosis (LL), slip angle (%), pelvic tilt (PT), thoracic kyphosis (TK). Reviewing the SDSG classification [13], we reasonably assumed a PT $\leq$ 30 degrees as a condition of pre- or post-operative balanced pelvis. In fact, as in the low than in the HGISL, the SDSG identified a balanced pelvis when the PT was $\leq 35°$, while the value $\geq 25°$ characterized an unbalanced pelvis. In this way, they produced a grey, borderline zone between 26° e 34°, in which the criteria of pelvic balance remain undefined. The median value of that gap is indeed 30°, which we have arbitrarily chosen as the separation point between balance and unbalance.

The study size is given by selection of the inclusion criteria. On the post-hoc estimated power tests the size of the sample was found to be excellent $(1- \beta) = 0.7$ (for α 0.05, effect size 0.8). The entire cohort was analyzed with SPSS v.18. ANOVA analysis was used to compare means of the investigated parameters between the two groups. Paired samples T-Tests were used to compare means of scores between pre- and postoperative radiological and clinical outcomes, Bivariate correlation were used for continuous variables (according to Pearson method), Univariate ANOVA and Repeated Measures ANOVA were used to compare means between the two subgroups. Threshold of statistical significance was considered to be $p < .05$.

All the patients of the surgical subgroup expressed consent to the surgical procedure after appropriate information. All the patients gave informed explicit consent to undergo the radiological follow-up, and were also elucidated about the purpose of this study. The local ethic committees of our Institutions had a favorable pronunciation about ethical issues because the study did not include a procedure which could provoke harm towards the individuals of the final cohort. No deviation from the generally recognized gold standard of care was performed on the patients. Moreover data reported have been completely anonymized. This study is perfectly consistent, in any of its aspect, with WMA Helsinki declaration of Human Rights.

3. RESULTS

Mean age was 24 (range 19-39), with F:M ratio 2.5:1. Seven deformities were type 7 (balanced pelvis) and 21 type 8 (unbalanced pelvis). The group A consisted of 2 type 7 and 12 type 8 deformities, while 5 type 7 and 9 type 8 established the group B. We recorded a total amount of 2 (7%) major early complications, related to a unilateral L5 nerve root palsy, completely recovered at 1 year, without neurological sequelae. Both patients belonged to the group A. Mean operative time was 187 min (range 150-220) in the group A and 205 (range 180-270) in the group B (p 0.05). Blood loss was significantly greater in the group A, as the postoperative hospital stay (8 ± 2 vs 4 ± 1 days) (p = 0.02). Mean blood loss was 550 (300-1200) in the group A versus 250cc (range 150-600) in the group B (p = 0.037). At the follow-up (mean 29,4; range 24-42), the improvement of slippage was 62% ± 3% in the group A and 65% ± 5% in the group B (p = 0.07). A patient of the group A was reoperated at 1 year to reduce a painful subcutaneous prominence of the right distal rod, without loss of the slip reduction. Post-operative changes of the spine and pelvis was summarized in Table 1. All patients with type 7 HGISL remained with a balanced pelvis, while the PT decreased below 30 degrees (from max 35° to min 22° on average; DS ± 4) in 9 type 8 HGISL (5 group A and 4 group B).

Slip angle improved about half from baseline in both groups (Figure 1 and 2), without substantial differences (p 0.07), while the L4-S1 LL slightly decreased (p 0.057). Two patients from groups (7%) showed a loss of the slip angle correction, due to intersomatic pseudoarthrosis but without breakage of the posterior implant (Figure 3). Indifferently, the SVA slightly increased in both groups (p 0.064). No substantial modifications suffered the TK between the groups (p > .05), although a declining trend was observed. Back and leg VAS, ODI and SF36 clearly improved from the baseline in either groups during the serial follow-up controls (Table 2). They were not affected by the pelvic modifications (Figure 4). The worst painful condition, considering mean back/leg VAS ≥ 6, was related to the degree of the slip angle: in 8 patients, a value > 10° appeared to have negative effects on the spinal health (p < .03) (Table 3).

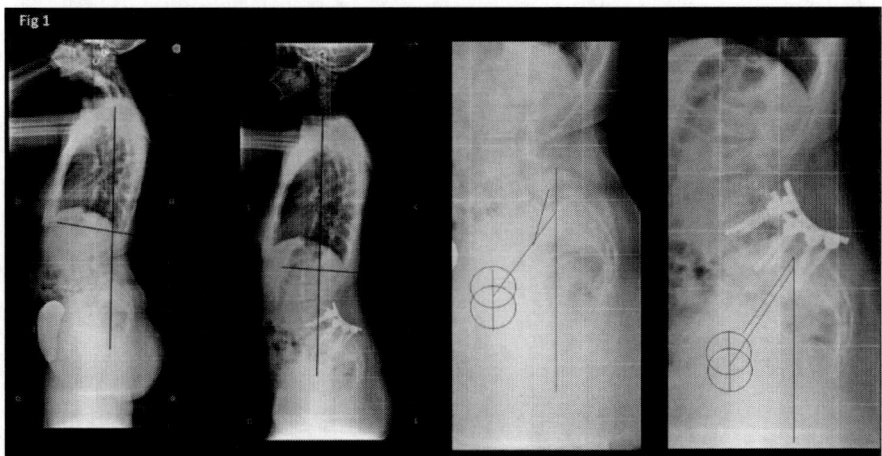

Figure 1. Type 8 HGISL operated by open surgery (Group A). a,b) Pre-operative and follow-up full spine standing x-rays showed a slight reduction of the LL and the forward displacement of the SVA; c,d) From the spino-pelvic point of view, the posterior instrumented fusion obtained a significant improvement of the slip angle (18° to 0°) and PT (32° to 25°).

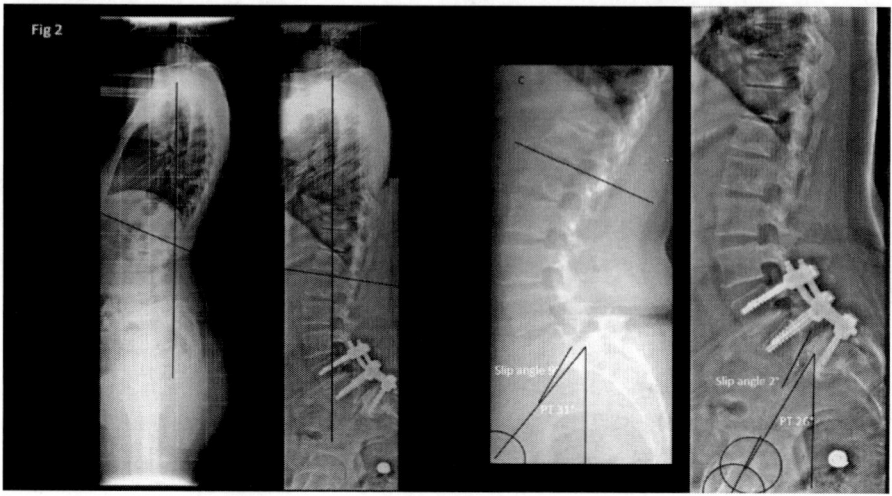

Figure 2. Type 8 HGISL mini-invasively treated (Group B). a,b) The comparison between pre-operative and follow-up full spine standing x-rays detected a small LL decrease and a SVA slipping forward; c,d) Slip angle and PT significantly decreased (respectively, 9° to 2° and 31° to 26°).

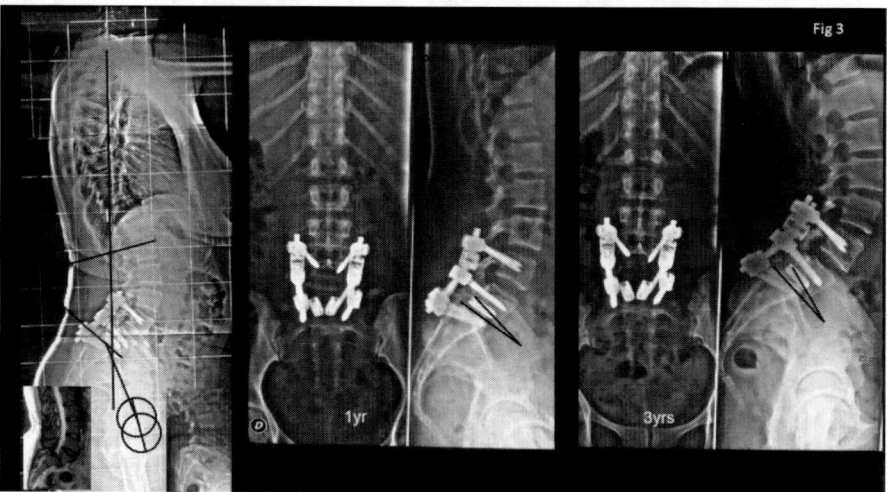

Figure 3. Type 8 HGISL (Group A) with loss of the slip angle correction. a) Three-years follow-up post-operative full spine standing x-ray (in the bottom, the pre-operative findings); b) At 1 yr follow-up, the slip angle was 8.5 degrees; c) The slip angle worsened up to 14° after 3 yrs. This condition was related to the worst painful follow-up condition (VAS back/leg 7).

Table 1. Summary in detail of the radiographic results of the groups A and B and statistical analysis within groups

HGISL (28 pts)	Mean SVA pre FU	Mean LL pre FU	Mean slip angle pre FU	Mean PT Pre FU	Mean TK Pre FU	p value
Group A (2 type 7)	0.8 (±1.2) 1.3 (±1)	58 (±7) 48 (±7)	16 (±8) 8 (±6)	26 (±3) 22 (±4)	35 (±10) 30 (±8)	<0.05
Group B (5 type 7)	0.6 (±1.5) 1 (±0.7)	55 (±8) 50 (±5)	13 (±8) 6 (±2)	35 (±4) 27 (±8)	38 (±5) 33 (±7)	<0.05
p value A vs B	0.064	0.057	0.07	0.06	0.057	

Table 2. Summary in detail of the mean clinical improvement in the group A and B and statistical analysis within groups

Mean values	VAS back Pre FU	VAS leg Pre FU	ODI (%) Pre FU	SF36 PCS (%) Pre FU	p value
Group A	8 3	7.3 3.8	55.6 39	27.6 40	.01 to .03
Group B	9 2.8	6.5 3.2	58.3 37.6	30 44.7	.01 to .03
p value A vs B	0.06	.076	0.067	0.07	

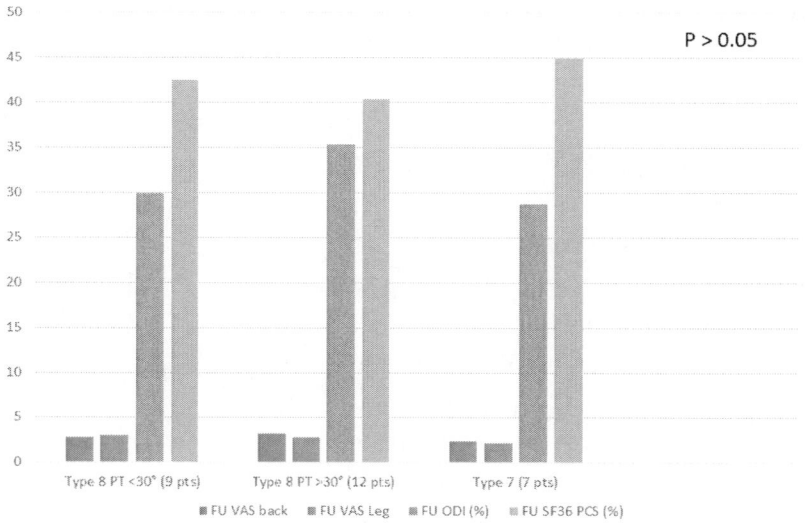

Figure 4. Post-operative pelvic changes and clinical outcomes: Graphical relationships and statistics (see the text).

Table 3. Follow-up back and leg VAS in patients with a slip angle lower or higher than 10°

Follow-up	Mean VAS back	Mean VAS leg
Slip angle > 10° (8pts)	5.3 (3-7)	4.2 (3-7)
Slip angle < 10° (20 pts)	3.5 (2-5)	2.5 (2-4)
p value	0.02	0.027

4. DISCUSSION

In the HGISL, surgery was indicated in symptomatic patients, with untreatable pain and/or radicular signs. In the lumbo-sacral junction, the proper surgical management remains still largely debated in literature [14, 15], especially for three surgical issues: the L5-S1 intersomatic fusion, L4 inclusion and percentage of slippage recovery. Nowadays, in situ fusion can be again debated [16], while anterior surgery seems affected by a high complication rate [17]. In this scenario, reduction and fusion by posterior pedicle screws, with or without intersomatic cages, has progressively achieved consensus [18, 19], but, to date, its effects on the spino-pelvic balance and clinical outcomes remain unclear [20, 21]. Recently the same groups of spinal surgeons reported that the reduction in high- to low-grade and normal pelvic balance may be the keys for a good QoL [22, 23]. The protocol of the present prospective investigation aims at immediately solving the first two aforementioned questions. In fact, in order to minimize the bias related to different surgical procedures, the final cohort included only patients who received a L4-S1 posterior instrumented fusion and L5-S1 PLIF. To realize fusion, we performed both open and MISS approach: to our knowledge, this is the first comparative study between an adult HGISL series mininvasively and another one invasively treated.

Literature lacks of data about the role of MISS in the treatment of HGISL, although few isolated case reports were referred as promising [8, 9]. Several studies were only focused on the rule of MISS-TLIF in the surgical treatment of low-grade isthmic spondylolisthesis, concerning pain resolution, functional outcomes, complications, fusion and revision rate[10,11].

A recent systematic meta-analysis on MISS-TLIF versus open surgery demonstrated that MISS was superior in reducing recovery and hospital stay length, but longer operative times were recorded [24]. We had similar results, except for the surgical time: it was not much longer in the MISS and predominantly related to the microscope setup and percutaneous operating procedure.

Regarding the issue about the real need for deformity correction, as described in unbalanced spine patients [25, 26] to restore a harmonic global alignment as well as possible, we always considered the reduction of the slippage. By performing open and MISS surgery, we achieved a partial incomplete slippage reduction, which should have allowed for the enough space to allocate the intersomatic cages, without increasing the risk for an excessive traction of the nerve roots, as recommended by some authors [21]. In the adult patients with a stiff spine, we believe that a partial slippage reduction may be approved and functioning for the interbody fusion, without intensifying the risk of neurological complications. Despite this caution, we recorded 2 (14%) L5 nerve palsy in the open group. Both surgical techniques seemed to have the same ability to correct the segmental deformity, improving slippage and slip angle, without changing the pelvic parameters in type 7 HGISL, but achieving a significant PT recovery $\leq 30°$ in over 40% of type 8 deformities. In practice, the surgical correction could result in modification from high- to low-grade and from type 8 to type 7. These radiographic results seem to confirm data by Alzakri et al. [22], collected from a series of adolescent spinal deformities treated by a posterior open surgery. By both surgical techniques adopted, LL and TK showed a mild decrease, while the SVA remained in the range of a balanced spine in all cases. Nevertheless, we noted some gentle forward displacement of the latter parameter, especially in cases with significant improvement of the PT. This SVA adaptation in the adult spine has never been detected by the literature: it may be a consequence of the post-surgical pelvic antiversion and TK decrease, with subsequent gradual forward compensation of the cervico-thoracic junction. At 2 years follow-up on average, these profile modifications did not have clinical consequences as the stiffness and/or pain of the low cervical spine.

Clinical evaluation was performed applying scores and questionaries universally accepted by the scientific spine community. Outcomes of the surgical treatments were significantly satisfactory, agreeing with the report by a recent prospective cohort study [27]. The VAS, ODI and SF-36 clearly improved from baseline, without differences between groups (p .06 to .08). Correlations between the clinical outcomes and spino-pelvic parameters surgical restoration were reported by Bourghli et al. [28] in patients affected by low-grade spondylolisthesis. The importance of the lumbar and pelvis shape on the QoL was also emphasized in an adult unoperated HGISL series [29]. Nevertheless, our experience lacks to confirm these literature data. Probably, the stable balanced spine manteined both before and after surgery could have decreased the fundamental rule of the pelvis in helping an asymptomatic condition. The spinal parameter that caused a worsening of pain was the slip angle, a specific measure of the L5 kyphosis: lack or failure of its correction, with value above 10°, affected our outcomes.

CONCLUSION

This study cannot lead to definitive findings. The main limitations lie in the exiguity of the sample and follow-up. Though a great effort has been made towards a rigorous methodology in patients eligibility, conclusions may suffer from under-representation bias. However the impact of many factors has been completely excluded, and the statistical power of the present comparison study remains high. In our hands, posterior surgery for the treatment of painful and intractable HGISL realized by open or MISS procedure was be able to guarantee radiographic and clinical results that seemed to maintain at 2 years follow-up. The MISS, with new advanced reduction instrumentations, showed some advantages in terms of short hospitalization and early recovery, as already reported in the treatment of other spinal pathologies. The search for correction by reduction screws and intersomatic cages, both in the presence or absence of a unbalanced pelvis, may improve the segmental deformity, decreasing the risk of implant mobilization and favoring the fusion. Slip angle value lower than 10 degrees seems to correlate with better clinical conditions.

Our observational study was based on a series of operated adult HGISL, divided into two homogeneous groups for demographic, clinical, radiological and surgical characteristics. Inclusion criteria were age >18yrs, L4-S1 posterior fusion, L5-S1 PLIF, balance of the spine. Data showed that the L4-S1 posterior approach may be overall feasible and effective in the treatment of HGISL. The MISS was *non inferior* in terms of clinical and radiological results but *superior* for an early post-operative recovery and hospital length. A key point was the bilateral insertion of PLIF-shaped cages that obtained a symmetric cantilever effect on the L5 inferior endplate, improving the slip angle. This angular value was crucial for our clinical outcomes. Further studies will be required to demonstrate a clear correlation between the radiological and clinical results. Our data showed that estimated parameters did not significantly affect the clinical outcomes as measured at the last follow-up, except for the slip angle.

REFERENCES

[1] Meyerding HW (1932) Spondylolisthesis: surgical treatment and results. *Surg Gynecol Obstet* 54:371–377.

[2] Wiltse LL, Newman PH, Macnab I (1976) Classification of spondylolysis and spondylolisthesis. *Clin Orthop* 117:23–29.

[3] Boxall D, Bradford DS, Winter RB, Moe JH (1979) Management of severe spondylolisthesis in children and adolescents. *J Bone Joint Surg* 61A(4):479–495.

[4] Marchetti PC, Bartolozzi P (1997) Classification of spondylolisthesis as a guideline for treatment. In: Bridwell KH, DeWald RL: *The textbook of spinal surgery, 2 ed.* Lippincott-Raven, Philadelphia pp 1211–1254.

[5] Roussouly P, Gollogly S, Berthonnaud E, Labelle H, Weidenbaum M (2006) Sagittal alignment of the spine and pelvis in the presence of

L5–S1 isthmic lysis and low-grade spondylolisthesis. *Spine* (Phila Pa 1976) 31:2484–2490.

[6] Labelle H, Mac-Thiong JM, Roussouly P (2011) Spino-pelvic sagittal balance of spondylolisthesis: a review and classification. *Eur Spine J* 20 (Suppl 5):641-45.

[7] Kasliwal MK1, Smith JS, Kanter A, Chen CJ, Mummaneni PV, Hart RA, Shaffrey CI (2012) Management of high-grade spondylolisthesis. *Neurosurg Clin N Am.* 24(2):275-91.

[8] Quraishi NA, Rampersaud YR (2013) Minimal access bilateral transforaminal lumbar interbody fusion for high-grade isthmic spondylolisthesis. *Eur Spine J* 22(8):1693–1699.

[9] Rajakumar DV, Hari A, Krishna M, Sharma A, Reddy M (2017): Complete anatomic reduction and monosegmental fusion for lumbar spondylolisthesis of Grade II and higher: use of the minimally invasive "rocking" technique. *Neurosurg Focus 43*(2):E12.

[10] Barbagallo G. M. V., Piccini M., Alobaid A., Al-Mutair A., Albanese V., Certo F (2014).: Bilateral tubular minimally invasive surgery for low-dysplastic lumbosacral lytic spondylolisthesis (LDLLS): Analysis of a series focusing on postoperative sagittal balance and review of the literature. *Eur Spine J.* 23:S705–S713.

[11] Wang J, Zhou Y, Zhang ZF, Li CQ, Zheng WJ, Liu J (2010) Comparison of one-level minimally invasive and open transforaminal lumbar interbody fusion in degenerative and isthmic spondylolisthesis grades 1 and 2. *Eur Spine J* 19:1780–1784.

[12] Mac-Thiong JM, Labelle H (2006): A proposal for a surgical classification of pediatric lumbosacral spondylolisthesis based on current literature. *Eur Spine J* 15:1425–1435.

[13] Mac-Thiong JM, Duong L, Parent S, Hresko MT, Dimar J, Weidenbaum M, Labelle H. (2012) Reliability of the SDSG classification of lumbosacral spondylolisthesis, *Spine* (Phila Pa 1976) 15;37(2):E95-102.

[14] Noorian S, Sorensen K, Cho W (2018) A systematic review of clinical outcomes in surgical treatment of adult isthmic spondylolisthesis. *Spine J.* 18(8):1441-1454.

[15] Transfeldt EE, Mehbod AA (2007) Evidence-based medicine analysis of isthmic spondylolisthesis treatment including reduction versus fusion in situ for high-grade slips. *Spine* (Phila Pa 1976) 32 (19 Suppl): S126–S129.

[16] Joelson A, Danielson BI, Hedlund R, Wretenberg P, Frennered K (2018) Sagittal Balance and Health-Related Quality of Life Three Decades After in Situ Arthrodesis for High-Grade Isthmic Spondylolisthesis. *J Bone Joint Surg Am.* Aug 15;100 (16):1357-1365.

[17] Alhammoud A, Schroeder G, Aldahamsheh O, Alkhalili K, Lendner M, Moghamis IS, Vaccaro AR. (2019) Functional and Radiological Outcomes of Combined Anterior-Posterior Approach Versus Posterior Alone in Management of Isthmic Spondylolisthesis. A Systematic Review and Meta-Analysis. *Int J Spine Surg.* Jun 30;13(3):230-238.

[18] Goyal N, Wimberley DW, Hyatt A, Zeiller S, Vaccaro AR, Hilibrand AS, Albert TJ (2009): Radiographic and clinical outcomes after instrumented reduction and transforaminal lumbar interbody fusion of mid and high-grade isthmic spondylolisthesis. *J Spinal Disord Tech* 22 (5): 321-327.

[19] Sears W (2005) Posterior lumbar interbody fusion for lytic spondylolisthesis: restoration of sagittal balance using insert-androtate interbody spacers. *Spine J* 5(2):161–169.

[20] Labelle H, Roussouly P, Chopin D, Berthonnaud E, Hresko T, O'Brien M (2008) Spino-pelvic alignment after surgical correction for developmental spondylolisthesis. *Eur Spine J* 17:1170–1176.

[21] Boachie-Adjei O, Do T, Rawlins BA (2002): Partial Lumbosacral Kyphosis Reduction, Decompression, and Posterior Lumbosacral Transfixation in High-Grade Isthmic Spondylolisthesis: Clinical and Radiographic Results in Six Patients. *Spine* 27(6):E161-E168.

[22] Alzakri A, Labelle H, Hresko MT, Parent S, Sucato DJ, Lenke LG, Marks MC, Mac-Thiong JM (2019) Restoration of normal pelvic balance from surgical reduction in high-grade spondylolisthesis. *Eur Spine J.* 28 (9): 2087-2094.

[23] Mac-Thiong JM, Hresko MT, Alzakri A, Parent S, Sucato DJ, Lenke LG, Marks M, Labelle H. (2019) Criteria for surgical reduction in

high-grade lumbosacral spondylolisthesis based on quality of life measures. *Eur Spine J.* 28 (9): 2060-2069.

[24] Wong AP, Smith ZA, Stadler JA 3rd, Hu XY, Yan JZ, Li XF, Lee JH, Khoo LT (2014) Minimally invasive transforaminal lumbar interbody fusion (MI-TLIF): surgical technique, long-term 4-year prospective outcomes, and complications compared with an open TLIF cohort. *Neurosurg Clin N Am.* Apr 25(2):279-304.

[25] Hresko MT, Labelle H, Roussouly P, Berthonnaud E (2007) Classification of high grade spondylolisthesis based on pelvic version and spinal balance: possible rationale for reduction. *Spine* 32(20):2208–2213.

[26] Labelle H, Roussouly P, Berthonnaud E, Dimnet J, O'Brien M (2005) The importance of spinopelvic balance in L5-S1 developmental spondylolisthesis: a review of pertinent radiologic measurements. *Spine* 30 (6 suppl):S27–S34.

[27] Bourassa-Moreau É, Labelle H, Parent S, Hresko MT, Sucato D, Lenke LG, Marks M, Mac-Thiong JM (2019) Expectations for Postoperative Improvement in Health-Related Quality of Life in Young Patients With Lumbosacral Spondylolisthesis: A Prospective Cohort Study. *Spine* (Phila Pa 1976) 44(3):E181-E186.

[28] Bourghli A, Aunoble S, Reebye O, Le Huec JC (2011): Correlation of clinical outcome and spinopelvic sagittal alignment after surgical treatment of low-grade isthmic spondylolisthesis. *Eur Spine J* (suppl 5):663–668.

[29] Gussous Y, Theologis AA, Demb JB, Tangtiphaiboontana J, Berven S (2018) Correlation Between Lumbopelvic and Sagittal Parameters and Health-Related Quality of Life in Adults With Lumbosacral Spondylolisthesis. *Global Spine J.* 8(1):17-24.

INDEX

A

adult spine deformity, 120
age, x, 14, 27, 59, 64, 106, 110, 120, 121, 124, 131
angiogenesis, 5, 26, 27, 29
ankylosing spondylitis, 17
anti-inflammatory drugs, 97
apoptosis, viii, 2, 13, 26, 27, 28, 29
arthrodesis, 27, 69, 79, 97, 98, 102
assessment, 9, 70, 71, 72, 73, 96
asymptomatic, 92, 97, 130

B

back pain, 6, 14, 15, 16, 18, 27, 61, 79, 94, 96, 121
beneficial effect, 25
bias, 123, 128, 130
bilateral, 16, 58, 60, 93, 98, 101, 103, 121, 131, 132
bioactive materials, 103
bioavailability, 24
biological markers, 24
biomarkers, 17
biomaterials, 36, 47
biomechanics, 84
bleeding, 26, 99, 109
blood, ix, x, 2, 3, 4, 21, 26, 37, 57, 66, 90, 104, 106, 108, 120, 124
blood clot, 2
blood transfusion, 66
blood vessels, 26
bone, vii, viii, 1, 3, 5, 8, 9, 10, 11, 12, 14, 16, 17, 18, 19, 25, 26, 27, 30, 40, 56, 57, 58, 60, 65, 68, 69, 70, 71, 73, 74, 75, 76, 78, 79, 80, 81, 82, 95, 97, 99, 101, 102, 103
bone form, 3, 26, 30, 71, 76, 102
bone growth, 18, 76
bone marrow, 9, 11, 12, 14, 16, 19, 25, 70, 99, 101, 103
bone marrow aspiration, 99, 101
bone resorption, 74

C

calcium, viii, 2, 56, 69, 78, 80, 95
cancer, 21, 30, 94, 105
cartilage, 12, 13, 27
cartilaginous, 102
Caucasian population, 91
cauda equina, 93, 97
cauda equina syndrome, 93, 97
cell death, 28, 29
cell signaling, 5
classification, 61, 62, 64, 70, 71, 72, 73, 74, 75, 84, 85, 92, 110, 113, 115, 122, 123, 132
claudication, 92, 93, 94, 105, 106
clinical application, 3, 31
clinical symptoms, 97
clinical trials, 9, 18, 31, 76
collagen, viii, 5, 6, 13, 14, 27, 56, 70, 76, 81
combination therapy, 20
communication, 20, 24, 59
complications, ix, x, 16, 18, 20, 26, 30, 61, 66, 76, 80, 90, 104, 109, 120, 123, 124, 128, 129, 134
compression, 93, 94, 103, 121, 122
controversial, ix, 17, 19, 89
correlation, x, 59, 77, 120, 123, 131
CT scan, vii, viii, 56, 59, 61, 62, 68, 69, 70, 71
culture, 13, 20, 30
culture medium, 30
current limit, 3, 10, 21
cytokines, 2, 5, 13, 28

D

data collection, 59
data set, 59
database, 24, 69
defects, 18, 80
deficiency, 93
deficit, ix, 90, 92, 94, 106, 109
degeneration, 6, 12, 13, 25, 27, 29, 32, 36, 38, 42, 46, 47, 49, 52, 75, 91, 93, 94
degenerative conditions, 69, 80
degradation, 24, 28
demonstrated, 5, 7, 8, 12, 14, 16, 57, 76, 129
diabetes, 26, 35, 36, 39, 40, 43, 47, 48, 51, 65
diabetic patients, 26, 31
diffusion-weighted imaging, 15
discs, 7, 8, 13, 14, 27, 28, 95
disease progression, vii, 1, 25
diseases, x, 17, 30, 31, 83, 113, 120
disk disease, 69, 85, 114, 115
displacement, 91, 125, 129
distribution, 92, 108

E

early recovery, 130
electrocautery, 101
electron microscopy, 23
embryonic stem cells (ESCs), 25
epidural hematoma, 84, 114
evidence, 3, 6, 9, 10, 12, 16, 18, 19, 21, 26, 30, 58, 70, 73, 75, 76, 77, 110, 111
extracellular matrix, viii, 2, 6, 13, 27, 28

F

fibrin, 102, 103
fibroblast growth factor, 5
fibroblast proliferation, 5
fixation, viii, 2, 15, 56, 60, 81, 84, 90, 111, 121, 122, 123
formation, 11, 26, 71, 72, 74
fusion, vii, viii, x, 5, 8, 15, 16, 19, 23, 25, 26, 31, 56, 57, 58, 59, 62, 66, 68, 69, 70, 71, 72, 73, 74, 75, 76, 77, 78, 79, 80, 81, 85, 87, 98, 101, 102, 104, 111, 114, 117,

120, 121, 123, 125, 128, 129, 131, 132, 133, 134
fusion rate, v, viii, 16, 25, 26, 31, 55, 56, 58, 59, 62, 68, 69, 70, 71, 76, 77, 78, 80, 81, 86, 115

G

ganglion, 85, 86, 115
ganglion cyst, 85, 86, 115
general anaesthesia, 60
general anesthesia, 98
genetic information, 21, 24
growth, viii, 2, 4, 5, 7, 9, 13, 18, 26, 76
growth factor, viii, 2, 4, 5, 7, 9, 76
guidance, 60, 98, 99, 103

H

healing, viii, 2, 3, 5, 8, 9, 11, 25, 27, 29
health, 29, 57, 125
height, 6, 13, 14, 15, 91, 102
herniated, ix, 7, 8, 90, 93, 104
herniated nucleus pulposus, 7, 8
hospitalization, ix, 57, 90, 104, 106, 108, 109
human, 8, 14, 16, 21, 26, 27, 80
hydroxyapatite, 70, 76, 80, 81
hypertrophy, 6, 75, 93

I

identification, 23, 60, 69
images, 61, 62, 68, 70, 71, 72, 73, 95
immobilization, 57, 75
immune response, 24
improvements, ix, 12, 14, 16, 26, 90
in vivo, 7, 8, 9, 12, 28
incidence, 26, 31, 76
individuals, 14, 121, 124

infection, 9, 20, 26, 27, 30, 60, 108, 109
inflammation, 2, 17, 29
inflammatory bowel disease, 17
injections, viii, 2, 3, 7, 13, 14, 15, 17, 18, 20, 24
injury, iv, 2, 57, 85, 115
insertion, 100, 102, 106, 109, 121, 131
internal fixation, 68
intervention, 6, 28, 106, 109
invasive spine surgery, 56, 108, 122
ipsilateral, 66, 98, 101, 102, 103
issues, 18, 30, 128
isthmic spondylolisthesis, iv, vi, vii, x, 64, 65, 78, 86, 115, 119, 120, 122, 128, 132, 133, 134

J

joints, 58, 72, 75, 81, 91, 94, 101

K

kyphosis, x, 80, 120, 123, 130

L

laminectomy, 60, 101
ligament, 2, 6, 58, 91, 101
lordosis, viii, x, 56, 57, 62, 77, 81, 91, 102, 103, 120, 122, 123
Lumbar Degenerative Spondylolisthesis (LDS), ix, 89, 90, 91, 92, 93, 94, 95, 97, 103, 105, 110, 111
lumbar spine, 14, 56, 61, 75, 80, 81, 91, 94, 110

M

major histocompatibility complex, 17, 18
management, 6, 85, 110, 114, 115, 128

manufacturing, 19, 30
materials, 60, 70, 76, 77, 81
matrix, viii, 5, 6, 7, 13, 28, 56, 60, 65, 81, 99, 101
matrix metalloproteinase, 13
measurement, 66, 67, 81
mesenchymal stem cells, 5, 8, 10, 25
microscope, 121, 129
migration, 12, 28, 76
minimally, iv, v, vi, vii, ix, 25, 37, 56, 76, 78, 80, 82, 84, 86, 89, 90, 97, 98, 100, 108, 111, 113, 115, 119, 120, 121, 122, 132, 134
Minimally Invasive - Transforaminal Lumbar Interbody Fusion (MI-TLIF), v, ix, 44, 89, 90, 98, 100, 103, 104, 105, 106, 108, 109, 111, 134
minimally invasive surgery, ix, 78, 90, 120, 121, 132
modifications, 66, 122, 125, 129
muscles, 85, 97, 99, 109, 115, 121
musculoskeletal, viii, 2, 3, 10, 12, 20, 26

N

nerve, 26, 58, 92, 93, 94, 101, 102, 121, 124, 129
non-steroidal anti-inflammatory drugs, 17
normal distribution, 105
nucleic acid, 22, 30
nucleotides, 22
nucleus, 6, 13, 27

O

observational study by prospective data, 122
ossification, 6, 57, 58, 73
osteoarthritis, 2, 9, 12
osteoclastogenesis, 26
osteoporosis, 8, 25, 26, 30, 59, 101

P

pain, vii, 1, 6, 7, 9, 12, 13, 14, 26, 27, 29, 57, 92, 93, 94, 96, 97, 99, 100, 103, 109, 121, 128, 129, 130
pelvis, x, 120, 123, 124, 130, 131
percutaneous pedicle screw fixation, 81, 90, 111
peripheral blood, 2, 11, 19
peripheral neuropathy, 27
permission, iv, 86, 87, 116, 117
phosphate, viii, 16, 56, 60, 65, 78, 79, 80
physical therapy, 27
physical treatments, 121
physicians, 20
plasma membrane, 21, 22, 24
plasticity, viii, 1, 10, 13
platelets, 2, 3, 4, 5
population, 13, 25, 94, 120, 122
posterior fusion, v, 72, 80, 89, 120, 131
post-operative, ix, 20, 30, 61, 67, 69, 81, 90, 100, 105, 109, 123, 124, 126, 127, 131
preparation, iv, 3, 5, 57, 58, 60, 102
proliferation, viii, 2, 5, 6, 7, 24, 25, 28
proteins, 21, 22, 23, 28, 30
proteolytic enzyme, 13
pseudarthrosis, 61, 62, 66, 67, 68, 69, 73, 74, 77
psoriatic arthritis, 17

Q

quality of life, 57, 85, 96, 97, 109, 114, 134
quiet, 76

R

radiculopathy, 3, 93, 94, 95, 105, 106
reconstruction, 12, 59, 61, 69, 72

recovery, ix, 14, 29, 90, 108, 109, 128, 129, 130, 131
regeneration, 5, 8, 12, 13, 18, 29
regenerative capacity, vii, 1, 11, 13
regenerative medicine, 21, 30
remodelled, 72
residual, 74, 75, 79
resolution, 86, 115, 128
response, 2, 13, 17, 18, 25, 76
restoration, 7, 57, 130, 133
risk, 25, 27, 30, 91, 103, 108, 129, 130
rods, 60, 98, 103, 104, 121, 122
root, ix, 90, 101, 102, 109, 121, 124
roots, 58, 93, 94, 109, 121, 129

S

safety, vii, ix, 15, 18, 80, 90
scoliosis, viii, 56, 63, 64, 66, 69, 80, 92
spinal cord injury, 20, 25
spinal fusion, 3, 10, 16, 25, 30, 75, 76, 77, 79, 81, 98
spinal stenosis, 6, 14, 85, 114
spine, iv, v, vii, 1, 3, 6, 8, 9, 10, 13, 14, 15, 17, 18, 20, 25, 26, 27, 31, 32, 33, 34, 36, 37, 38, 39, 40, 41, 42, 43, 44, 45, 46, 47, 48, 49, 50, 52, 53, 56, 57, 59, 61, 63, 72, 75, 78, 79, 80, 81, 82, 83, 84, 85, 86, 87, 91, 94, 103, 108, 109, 110,111, 112, 113, 114, 115, 116, 117, 120, 121, 122, 123, 124, 125, 126, 129, 130, 131, 132, 133, 134
spondylolisthesis, vii, viii, x, 6, 56, 64, 69, 70, 78, 79, 92, 100, 102, 110, 111, 120, 122, 128, 130, 131, 132, 133, 134
stabilization, viii, 2, 95, 97, 98, 103, 104, 106, 108
standard deviation, 64, 105, 107
stem cells, viii, 2, 10, 12, 18, 19, 24, 27
stenosis, ix, 16, 69, 90, 92, 93, 95, 98, 101, 104, 105, 106

subcutaneous tissue, 99
surgery, iv, vii, ix, 1, 2, 8, 9, 12, 16, 18, 25, 26, 27, 32, 34, 37, 38, 39, 40, 43, 44, 46, 47, 48, 51, 55, 59, 61, 63, 64, 67, 68, 69, 70, 71, 75, 76, 82, 84, 85, 87, 89, 96, 97, 98, 105, 106, 107, 108, 112, 113, 114, 116, 121, 122, 123, 125, 128, 129, 130, 131
surgical, viii, ix, x, 2, 15, 27, 29, 31, 36, 46, 47, 56, 57, 60, 65, 66, 74, 79, 81, 85, 86, 89, 90, 91, 92, 94, 96, 97, 98, 99, 100, 101, 103, 108, 109, 111, 114, 115, 116, 120, 122, 124, 128, 129, 130, 131, 132, 133, 134
surgical intervention, 27
surgical technique, 57, 74, 79, 129, 134
surgical techniques, 57, 129
symptoms, 13, 17, 27, 94, 97, 121

T

target, viii, 2, 12, 13, 21, 24
techniques, 21, 23, 30, 56, 57, 71, 76, 78, 81, 97, 108, 111, 129
therapeutic benefits, 24
therapeutic effect, 24
therapeutics, 21, 30
therapy, 10, 12, 14, 17, 18, 19, 29, 31
tissue, vii, ix, 1, 2, 5, 11, 19, 24, 28, 90, 98, 100, 101, 103, 121
titanium, viii, 56, 60, 65, 66, 78
transforming growth factor, 5
treatment, vii, viii, ix, x, 2, 7, 10, 12, 13, 14, 15, 17, 18, 19, 21, 25, 26, 27, 28, 29, 30, 31, 56, 57, 79, 80, 82, 85, 90, 94, 96, 97, 103, 107, 110, 111, 114, 120, 122, 128, 130, 131, 132, 133, 134

V

vascular endothelial growth factor (VEGF), 5

W

wires, 99, 101, 103
worldwide, 25, 26, 27
wound healing, 2, 5, 27, 30
wound infection, 66